With appreciation and love

to Hazel

at Christmas, 1982

from

Miriam Wood

Though He Slay Me

Though He Slay Me

A story of courage shining through heart-aches such as few of us have experienced

Miriam Wood

Review and Herald Publishing Association
Washington, D.C. 20012

Editor: Thomas A. Davis
Book Design: Alan Forquer
Cover: Harry Knox Associates; Gary Huff

Library of Congress Cataloging in Publication Data

Wood, Miriam.
Though he slay me.

1. Jefferson, Helen. 2. Jefferson, Stanley.
3. Seventh-day Adventists—United States—Biography. 4. Huntington's chorea—Patients—United States—Biography. I. Title.
BX6191.W66 286.7'3 [B] 81-10596
ISBN 0-8280-0102-2 AACR2

ACKNOWLEDGMENT

The words and music of the song "The Healer of Broken Hearts" (p. 322) are by Georgia Stiffler, © copyright 1945, © copyright renewed 1971 by Fred Bock Music Co., owner, Box 333, Tarzana, California 91356. All rights reserved. Used by permission.

Printed in U.S.A.

This book is prayerfully
DEDICATED
to every Christian who has been called upon
to suffer
extraordinary sorrow.

CONTENTS

PROLOGUE

THIS is the story of one woman's extraordinary courage in the face of a lifetime of adversity. From the invalidism of her mother when she was a child, through her lonely young-girl years when she was away from home in an unsympathetic environment, to the early years of her marriage when life was a round of constant drudgery, lack of money, and high expectations of her on the part of others, to the tragedy of her husband's long illness, Helen has faced whatever has come with faith in God, determination, energy, and a remarkable sense of humor.

She does not consider herself an unusual person in any way. She would scoff at the faintest suggestion that she is. Yet those who know her best are aware of the depths of her faith, the reality of her dependence upon God. It is one thing to face the sudden death of a husband—and it is a searing blow. But nothing in the lexicon of human experience can be more bruising to the spirit than the hopeless, long-continued, and deteriorating illness of a marriage partner. When the direction can only be downward, and yet life must be lived, hour by hour, day by day, the human spirit faints under the load. Only those who have survived such an experience can really empathize and understand.

There is no more cruel disease than Huntington's chorea, which was Stan's fate. The fact that it is working its deadly schemes in the body for years before it is detected is one of its more bitter features. The patient is thought of as merely intransigent, ugly of disposition, determined to hurt those around him. He is treated for a variety of scattered symptoms. It is only after a certain length of time has elapsed that those who love him finally learn the truth—the truth that they can never really accept, the truth that asserts that the loved one will sink to a level of animal existence as the years progress. And yet death does not come directly from the disease. It is usually the result of other complications resulting from poor circulation, poor nutrition, or other factors.

Of the disease *Encyclopedia Americana,* International Edition, 1976, says,

> Huntington's Chorea leads to progressive disability and death. It is a rare . . . disease. It starts in middle life, usually with a few scattered jerking moments or minor defects in coordination. The disease progresses gradually, and within a few years the jerks become grotesque and violent, and finally disabling. In almost every case, mental deterioration soon develops, producing memory loss, emotional outbursts, slovenly behavior, and severe dementia. . . . Extensive degenerative changes develop in many portions of the cerebral cortex and areas deep within the brain, but the precise nature of the underlying biochemical disorder is unknown. *No therapy will halt the progress of Huntington's Chorea.*

The description of the course of the disease in *RN,* August, 1977, seems as though it had been written with Stan Jefferson in mind:

> H.D. is a degenerative disorder of the central nervous system. Premature degeneration of nerve tissue in the cerebral cortex and at the basal ganglia from unknown causes brings on the major symptoms of the disease: personality changes, mental deterioration, and movement disorders. The disease is progressive, culminating in total incapacity and death, usually from superimposed infection. . . . H.D. usually shows up in the third or fourth decade of life and is insidious; a quiet, gentle person becomes tense with outbursts of temper; an excitable person becomes passive and withdrawn. Symptoms such as irritability, restlessness, confusion, poor recent memory, impaired judgment, and carelessness may appear. Motor disturbances often show up first as facial tics and progress to distorted grimaces. . . .

> Eventually spasmodic jerking movements of the muscles of the face, tongue, neck, trunk, and extremities take control of the victim, impairing balance and preventing locomotion. As the disease progresses, speech becomes hesitant or explosive and finally incoherent; swallowing becomes increasingly difficult, leading to frequent choking episodes; and the patient loses bowel and bladder control.

From the *American Journal of Nursing,* August, 1979, comes this horrifying description:

> The onset is insidious. Problem solving concept formation, verbal storage, alertness, and concentration are impaired. Mental deterioration is progressive, and impulsive behavior may cause such social problems as alcoholism, drug addiction, and sexual promiscuity. With progressive loss of intellect, the person becomes unable to carry on daily-living tasks and finally he becomes completely dependent.
>
> The difficulty in thinking and communicating interferes with expressing needs and fears, which contributes to feelings of social isolation. Emotional disturbances may result from distress over prognosis and difficulties in adjusting to a generally lower level of adaptive abilities.
>
> Paranoid delusions, grandiose ideas, and hallucinations may be described, and depressed states with suicidal tendencies are not uncommon. . . .
>
> Choreic movements, which are jerky, irregular, and stretching, usually appear first in the face, neck, and arms. Continuous involuntary movements of the facial and tongue muscles give rise to grotesque grimacing, clucking sounds, and a peculiar speech that eventually becomes unintelligible. Irregular movements of the trunk are present; the gait is shuffling and dancing. The upper body seems to advance ahead of the pelvis and legs, with the trunk assuming a rocking movement and the arms swinging from side to side. As the disease progresses, walking becomes impossible and swallowing difficult.

Huntington's chorea is, quite simply, more than a human being should ever be called upon to endure. The victim suffers excruciatingly. Those who love him suffer more.

New medications are proving helpful in controlling the grimaces and other symptoms of the disease, and at the present time more and more research is being conducted around the world in reference to this.

It is impossible to describe the panic that overwhelms a wife who sees the husband to whom she is closer than anyone else in the world becoming a stranger whom she does not know. One cannot put into words the thousand hurts, the humiliations, the fear, the utter hopelessness of it all.

Helen and Stan were friends of mine at Pacific Union College. I admired them both. As the years went by, I was aware that Stan was considered "up and coming" and was unusually successful in the ministry. Then came the sad news that he had renounced his commitment to God and had disappeared from Helen's life. At that point no one was aware that he was in the grip of an incurable illness. Helen suffered every anguish, shed every tear that is the lot of a wife who has been abandoned and "disgraced." Only much later did it become clear that Stan was not responsible for his actions.

If I were merely telling a story, I would not choose to tell this one, for there is so much heartache involved. But I believe with every fiber of my being that Helen's story can give courage to every human being who must endure the unendurable, who must bear the unbearable. Her love for Stan, her triumph over circumstances, and her unwavering faith in God are beacon lights in a dark world.

I have, of course, protected Stan as best I could. Even though the disease stripped him of nearly every shred of personhood, he was still a human being, a child of God. It is totally unnecessary to describe all his sufferings, all his humiliations.

It is my hope that this affirmation of faith will create more faith in the heart of every reader.

Miriam Wood

Though He Slay Me

CHAPTER 1

Beginnings

SOMETHING was different. Something was strange and frightening. The tiny brown-haired girl crept closer to her parents' bedroom door, closed and forbidding. Behind it she could hear the murmur of voices. The doctor had been in there such a long time. And she was sure she'd heard her mother crying. Maybe if she sat very, very quietly and listened, everything would be all right again. Her mother wouldn't be sick, as she'd been for so many weeks, and her father would be laughing as he always did, his curly red hair gleaming in the sunlight, his pince-nez glasses sparkling.

Then words began to take shape as she pressed against the wall, words that to the child sounded the end of the happy, secure world she'd known.

"What will we do? What will happen to us?" Her mother's voice was strained and tired. "Helen is only 3 years old; she needs to be taken care of all the time. And the two older boys . . . Oh, how could I have gotten tuberculosis? How could I?"

The child had heard enough. She turned and fled into the bright sunshine of the Nevada day, running, running, running, until the familiar sights of Reno restored a measure of security. After all, there was still the little house she lived in, still the sidewalk running by, still her grandmother's house across the street, and the vast reaches of the desert in the distance. Everything would be all right.

But the three people in the small bedroom were facing a grim future.

"Mr. Sanford," the kindly family doctor said, "your wife must be in bed most of the time. She must never, under any circumstances, do any work. Fortunately, the desert air here in Reno is favorable for tuberculosis—for recovery. But total rest is the only known treatment."

Slow tears coursed down the frail young woman's face. Seeing them, her tall, vital husband swept her into his arms.

"Don't you worry, sweetheart," he whispered. "It's going to be all right. We'll work it out."

"But how?" was her despairing question.

"Let me think," he told her. "But for now, just you lie there and stay comfy, and don't you worry."

She gave him a watery smile.

On the porch, the two men continued their discussion, their faces grave. Helen, seeing her father, ran to him and clasped him around the legs, looking into his face with eager expectation.

"Daddy, is Mommy sick?" she wanted to know.

"I'll tell you all about it later, Helen," he told the child.

"Mr. Sanford, I can't emphasize too strongly what I told both of you earlier. Mrs. Sanford's very life depends upon her complete rest. And if she is going to remain here at home for the time being, as you have indicated that you wish her to do, then her linens and dishes must be kept separate from those used by other members of the family. And she must have good, nourishing food—as much of it as you can coax her to eat."

As the doctor walked out to his car, the tall red-haired young father picked up his little girl. She burrowed her face into his shoulder. Everything really would be all right. Daddy would make it all right. He always had.

But her father's thoughts were turbulent, apprehensive. If only Etta hadn't worked so hard for the war effort, if only she hadn't felt that she had to help the United States win the war single-handedly. Nineteen eighteen will always be bordered in black for our family, he thought. But there was no time for philosophy or for regrets. Decisions had to be made, plans had to be constructed.

"Now, Helen," he said firmly, "I want you to go over to Aunt Clara's house and stay there until I call you for supper." Putting her down, he gave her an encouraging little pat, which elicited a smile over her shoulder. She was used to spending lots of time with Aunt Clara and her cousin Dorothea; Mother had had what she heard the adults call "the flu" for several weeks. "The flu" seemed to be part of everyone's vocabulary. Helen knew it was bad and it made everyone sick and some people cried and there were flowers.

Mr. Sanford went into the kitchen and sat down at the clean table. The past rolled through his mind as though it were on a never-ending screen. He remembered the pretty young woman he had met, a young woman with a broken marriage behind her and a little boy to support. She had been a cashier in a dry-goods store, brilliant, sparkling, and fiercely independent. Surely their first meeting couldn't have been more inauspicious. He'd been the grand master at a dance to which she'd agreed to go with friends. But when she got there she wouldn't dance, even though, after proper introductions had been made, he'd begged and begged her to be his partner.

"She didn't tell me that she'd attended that strange Seventh-day Adventist church as a little girl and picked up their weird ideas about not dancing and smoking and all the rest," he said to himself, smiling. "I just thought she wasn't interested in me." He had persisted doggedly in his determination to get to know her. Finally, near the end of the evening, she turned to him and declared, "If you knew all about me, you wouldn't spend any more time with me!"

Instantly he had replied, "I'll bet you a hole in a doughnut that there's nothing anyone could tell me about you that would make me not want to see you again!"

Later she told him that although she certainly was attracted to him, she didn't expect to see him again, for in the early 1900s not many women were divorced; it was assumed that those who were had brought their predicament on themselves and that they would be very poor marriage prospects. But he was undiscouraged. He didn't have red hair for nothing.

The next day he'd appeared at noon at the dry-goods store carrying a sack of "doughnut holes" that he'd wheedled the local baker into selling him. Very ceremoniously he presented this bag to Henrietta—actually, "Etta," as she was always known. He remembered her momentary disbelief as she opened the bag and realized the significance of the gift.

For two years the courtship progressed, steadily. "I really had to court both Etta and Harry," he remembered, "for he certainly was part of the bargain." And then there was the marriage, and the next year blond Marvin was born. Always Etta had been like a whirlwind of energy and enthusiasm, even through her own peritonitis and the boys' scarlet fever at Helen's birth.

He roused from his reverie as he heard her calling, her voice weak—so unlike her.

"We've had a good time together, haven't we?" she asked him wistfully.

"Well, of course we have—and we're going to have more good times! Don't talk as though it's all over!" he exclaimed.

She was silent for a moment. "But we have to face that possibility," she said quietly.

And they both remained silent, with thoughts too deep for tears. Then she regained some of her old sparkle.

"I'll never forget how upset your mother was when she heard that you were going to marry a Reno divorcée," she smiled.

"Nor how delighted Father was with you when he came to visit us after Mother's death," he smiled back. "He always said if Mother had only known you, she would have been so happy. I wish she had known that we named Helen for her."

His face set into unhappy lines. "I also wish that when Father died and left me the insurance money, I hadn't lost my head. I don't know what got into me. I was spending money as though it were water—and if I'd just saved it, with my job we'd be able to manage fine."

She put her hand on his. "Don't blame yourself, Ben. You've always been so generous and kind. And don't forget that we did buy this little house and though it may not be very grand, at least it's all ours."

"And it certainly was a bargain for only $1,650, when you consider that all the dishes and linens and household goods were included—even a pump organ. And then when Father Sanford gave us his lovely silver, crystal, and Haviland china, we really were fortunate," he agreed. "But I want you to sleep for a while, and when you wake up, I'll have a nice supper for you and the children."

"Are you sure that——" but he put his hand gently across her mouth and gave her shoulder a squeeze.

For small Helen, the changes came so thick and fast she could hardly comprehend them all. Now it was Daddy who got the three children up each morning, fed them and her mother, got the two boys off to school, and sent Helen to Aunt Clara's before seven-thirty when he left for work.

It was Grandma who gave Helen her baths; sick and almost helpless as she was, Etta Sanford was determined that her little girl should be taught modesty. To be bathed by her father would not have fitted her conception of modesty, a standard common in those times. So the lively, sturdy little girl looked forward to bathtimes with Grandma. It was Daddy, though, who tucked her in bed each night with a tender kiss.

And then there was Sarah, who came once a week to give the house a good cleaning—Sarah, with her black skin and loving heart, who became a part of the family.

"Daddy, what are 'poor white trash'?" Helen asked her father one night as he tucked her in.

Startled, he responded, "Why in the world do you want to know that?"

"Because the neighbor lady said we're 'poor white trash' 'cause Sarah eats at the table with us," Helen told him.

From her bed, Helen's mother overheard the conversation.

"That's a terrible thing for any human being to say about another human being," she declared. "God created all people equal, and as long as Sarah works in our home she will eat with us just as anyone else would," she told her. "Skin color has nothing to do with anything."

Life was a very grim struggle for the young father, though he was determined that his children should be as little aware of it as possible. He knew that they could not be protected from all the hardships of an invalid mother, but he hoped that their childhood would not be scarred forever. Helen was his special worry, his special heartache. A little girl needs a mother.

Ben Sanford was a charming, well-groomed, affectionate man who never realized his full potential because he lacked education. A serious eye problem as a child had kept his schooling to a minimum, and a serious accident to his neck had kept him in bed for two years. With no skills and no training, he finally became a meat cutter, a job he worked at sometimes twelve hours a day in a small grocery store several blocks from the house. To his children he was demonstrative and loving.

Etta Sanford was made of somewhat sterner stuff. She loved her children, but seldom found herself able to express her love as tangibly as Ben did. She was prone at times to see their faults rather than their virtues. She was determined that the lessons she had learned in her own hard life would be transmitted to them. Born when her mother was only 16, she had had to care for younger children after her father died when she was 13, and the iron of poverty and deprivation had entered deeply into her soul.

Helen turned to her father for the love and care both circumstances and temperament prevented her mother from giving her. A tremendous feeling of insecurity, of fear of the unknown, grew in the child's heart and mind when her world was turned topsy-turvy. Mother must not be bothered; Aunt Clara was busy with her family and problems; Grandmother, whom she adored, was busy every moment with her mother and the house and meals. Only when her highchair stood beside her father's chair at suppertime and he mashed her potatoes and cut her meat for her did the little girl feel that the world was a safe and friendly place to be. (Of course Ben Sanford spoiled his little daughter; how could he help it?)

"Now, children," their father said to them, soon after the tuberculosis was discovered, "just because your mother is sick is no excuse to let things go around here. We are going to run a really tight ship. Everything is going to be kept neat and tidy. The kitchen is always going to be clean, and the dishes are going to be kept washed. And each of you will keep your toys put away."

They did as they were told. The house was neat, though perhaps not as neat as Etta Sanford's critical eye might have wished. As a young teen, she had worked as a domestic in various wealthy homes and had absorbed from those experiences standards of cleanliness and beauty that she retained all her life. Before her illness she scrubbed and polished endlessly and relentlessly, beating back the determined desert sand as though it were a mortal enemy. She seemed never to understand that when she had worked as a domestic, the people for whom she had worked had done nothing for themselves. Now she filled the role of both employer and "employee." Her standards were almost impossibly high, and as the years went on and compromise with those standards had to be made, the trauma to her was very great.

Helen drifted from her house to her aunt's house, sometimes like a little wraith. Seeing her struggling with her little clothes and taking care of herself, the young father's heart would turn sad. There were never enough hours in the day, never enough dollars to meet the bills, never enough of anything to "go around." But he comforted himself that Helen, too, had spunk—in fact, she sometimes showed so much spunk that he knew she'd eventually get into some difficulties! Surely life would be kind to his little girl.

For Helen, the high point of the day arrived just before six o'clock when she walked the six long blocks to "Daddy's store" and walked home with him. If she craftily arrived a bit early, he would often slip her a piece of candy and whisper conspiratorially, "Now don't tell Mamma!" Helen didn't, but she paid for the sweets with cavities in her molars when she was still a little girl. It was a small price to pay for that special closeness with Daddy.

When she was only 4, her mother called her to her bed and declared, "Helen, it is time that you learned to embroider. Now go over to the bottom drawer of my dresser and bring me that square of cloth you'll find and the embroidery thread and the hoops and the scissors."

Excited, Helen ran to get the needed objects. Then she perched on the bed, ready to launch into a whole new world, sure that she would conquer it in short order. Alas for her expectations! The first lesson, a running stitch, looked so simple. But the thread kept getting tangled, and Mother kept commanding relentlessly, "Take the stitches out and start over." Finally Helen was in tears of frustration and fatigue. But the next day there was another lesson, and finally the running stitch became manageable. But that was only the beginning, for then she had to tackle the "lazy daisy" stitch, which involved looping the thread around the needle. Helen's small fingers were scarred with pricks from her needle, and her self-confidence bruised with the never-ending command, "Take the stitches out and start over."

But finally her first little bit of embroidery was finished. Looking it over critically, her mother declared, "Well, Helen, I guess this will do. Now I'm going to keep this for you, and when you are a grown woman you'll have the first embroidery you ever did." Helen, released from her torment, cared very little about the preservation of the work of art.

She was afraid of so many things. She was afraid of the dark. She was afraid of high places. She was afraid that something would happen to her mother—something worse than had already happened. She was afraid of the house where everyone must be quiet and let Mother rest and where everything must be kept picked up and where she heard her parents discussing finances at night when they thought she was asleep.

When she was about 5, the word *mortgage* first entered her world in an overheard conversation between her parents.

"There's no other way," her father had declared. "To meet our doctor bills, we will have to mortgage the house."

Her mother had gasped. "But it's the only thing we have! It's paid for. As long as we have it, we have a roof over our heads for our children. Isn't there any other way?"

Sadly Ben had replied, "None that I can think of."

Helen didn't know what a mortgage was and she was afraid to ask. But it was one more frightening thing in her unsettled world.

Then there were the Indians whom she saw on the streets of Reno. With the reservation only about a mile away, they came into town every day and would sit for hours on the sunny sidewalks. The squaws would unwrap the babies and sun them, while Helen crept timidly by, as far from the Indians as she could get. They were so strange. They were so different. What were they thinking, behind their opaque eyes and expressionless faces?

When the next-door neighbor hired an Indian squaw to do her washing, Helen was terrified. Each Monday she tried to stay as far from Mrs. Nelson's as possible, but on one dreadful Monday she was trapped. She had to walk right by the Indian woman, whose name, she had discovered, was "Mattie."

Gasping with relief, she rushed to her mother's bed. "I walked right by Mattie, and she didn't even bite me!" she exclaimed.

Annoyed, her mother replied, "Helen, where in the world do you get the foolish ideas you come up with? Mattie doesn't bite. No Indian bites, any more than we bite."

Helen wasn't convinced. She wasn't convinced that one could safely climb high places, either. But there was a hill not far away on which grew the most beautiful wildflowers. Helen, whose love for flowers was passionate and compulsive, longed to gather some of them. But there was a bridge to cross that seemed to her eyes as high as the sky.

Her grandmother said one day, "Helen, I'll take you for a walk. We'll go up on the hill and pick some of the flowers I've heard you praise so much."

Helen's blue eyes opened wide. "But we'll have to cross the river on that old footbridge," she whispered tremulously.

"But it's just a bridge, and it's completely safe. Now let's not hear another word about it" was her grandmother's brisk rejoinder.

As the two of them neared the bridge, Helen's heart beat so fast she thought she would choke. She couldn't bear to look down. She just put one small foot in front of the other and finally—after an eternity—they were across.

"Now that wasn't bad at all, was it?" her grandmother demanded.

Helen gulped. It was very bad, she thought, but she didn't want to seem sassy. Later that night she heard Grandmother talking to her father.

"I can't for the life of me understand why Helen is afraid of so many things. I thought I might have to carry her across that bridge today. You know it's as safe as a rocking chair."

Her father answered quietly, "A little girl whose mother is sick may not see things quite as they are."

And so a year went by, and then another, and Etta Sanford's condition seemed to remain about the same.

Sometimes she would have a surge of strength and be able to be up for short periods. As she lay in her lonely bed, with the household sounds around her and despair in her heart at the needs of her husband and children, she began to think of God and the religion she'd heard about when she lived with her Aunt Henrietta. The latter was a very cold and cruel woman, who had worked her unmercifully and not thought of sending her to an Adventist academy, even though, till her father died, she had been at the head of her class. Her aunt was a heavy contributor to the Seventh-day Adventist Church. When Etta's aunt had thrown down the gauntlet and "dared" her to be baptized, she had promptly done so—but with no comprehension of what was involved, or no intention of living by the tenets of the church. But the seeds were there and had lain dormant for many years.

Just before she had contracted tuberculosis, with World War I raging, she had suddenly felt a deep longing for a church home. But where could she go? She remembered the humble little Adventist church not far from her house, but the very sight of it annoyed her.

"I am telling you one thing," she informed her husband. "I think we should teach the children some religion, but I absolutely *will not* have them saddled with those Seventh-day Adventist beliefs, especially that old Adventist Sabbath!"

"Anything you want to do is all right with me," he told her.

After more thought she decided that the family would attend the Episcopalian church, since Ben had been reared in that faith and had been an altar boy. It was the church of the upper class; it was "respectable." There would be just enough religion and no meddling with everyday life. She made her careful plans, togged the children out in their best clothes, and, with the children's eyes wide with the unaccustomed experience, they entered the dignified church. They were escorted to a pew. The church building was gracious. The congregation was prosperous. The music was beautiful. Then the preacher stood up.

Stepping to the podium, he read the story of Creation in a resounding, melodious voice. Etta nodded, enjoying the sound of the familiar words. The preacher then turned around, very ceremoniously put the Bible on a table behind him as though dusting his hands of it, and announced, "We now know that science has disproved this ridiculous story."

It was too much for Etta Sanford. All unsuspected by her, the doctrinal teachings of Adventism had taken root more deeply than she had imagined. She never went back to the Episcopal church—but neither would she attend the Adventist church.

Then, lying in her bed one day, she called her husband. "Don't faint—but I want the children to have some religion. I know we didn't keep up with the Episcopal Church—and I know I've said lots of negative things about the Adventist Church. I've even studied the Jehovah's Witnesses material, but they use their own ideas, not the Bible. So if it's all right with you, I'd like for them to go to the Adventist Sabbath school."

Surprised, he replied, "Well, you know I've never objected to anything you wanted to do along that line."

Helen and Harry and Marvin went to Sabbath school. They didn't know any of the children there, and they didn't know what was expected of them, but Helen especially tried to fit in. If Mother thought she should go, there must be a good reason, even though the whole thing was totally mystifying.

CHAPTER 2

Growing and Working

HELEN and her two older brothers were introduced to the world of adult responsibility at a very early age. The slender resources of the family were dwindling away with alarming rapidity. Grandma could manage only so much work, though she spent her full time in their home. The washing alone was a staggering task. Obviously she could not cook the meals, supervise the children, change the invalid's bed every day, do the grocery buying, and still scrub the linens and personal clothing for the family on a washboard in a galvanized tub. So money had to be found to send the laundry to a "wet wash," a practice at that time. The clothes came back wet; they had to be hung on the line; the shirts had to be starched; all the clothing, pillowcases, and sometimes sheets (depending on the standards of the housewife) had to be sprinkled down and ironed the next day. Life was not easy for women.

Helen's childhood was short-lived. Her small hands were put at any task that her grandmother felt that she could manage—and sometimes at tasks that were beyond her maturity level. But the little girl absorbed the philosophy that she must always cope, she must always manage. She must never say "I can't," because there simply was no one else to take over. Dimly she remembered the first three years of her life when it had all been so different. Sometimes, during lonely afternoons, playing with her cousin Dorothea, she would declare, "When I'm a mommy I'm never going to be sick, and nobody in my house is ever going to be sick!" If people could just stay well, she thought, nothing else would matter. The conviction grew in small Helen that if she could just "catch" the tuberculosis from her mother, then the latter would be well again. Her childish mind did not pursue the thought of what might happen to her own body; it would be enough, she thought, if only her mother could be gloriously well again.

Flowers of all kinds were her solace. She helped with her grandmother's brave plantings in the dry, hard soil, watering the seeds lovingly. She picked wildflowers. The neighbors, who took a compassionate interest in the sturdy, lonely little girl, soon learned that to give Helen a flower was to bring brightness to her day.

Suddenly it was time for Helen to enroll in school.

"Now, Helen," her mother told her, having called her into the bedroom, "I expect you to do your best and to behave yourself and do exactly what your teacher tells you. I will not have a little girl who gets in trouble at school."

All the insecure feelings and just-below-the-surface fears came together in one throat-stopping ball. Helen was afraid of strangers. Her mother's illness had prevented the family from entertaining in their home; they were never invited to the homes of others, for the same reason, so that her world was bounded by family and the neighbors on her street. But what were other people like? What would happen in school?

"I've been embroidering little aprons for you to wear over your dress each day," her mother said. "I want you to look clean and nice all the time and to keep your clothes in good order."

Helen gazed at the pretty little aprons silently.

The first day of school was a kaleidoscope of faces, sounds, sensations. Of course Harry and Marvin had given dire predictions and lofty assessments of the teachers in the public school so close to their home. They'd relished the fear and uncertainty on Helen's face, never realizing, with the unconcern of childhood, that she needed their reassurance.

However, Helen's teacher, Miss Benjamin, was an understanding and outgoing woman. She gathered the child into her warm and outgoing personality. Helen felt that she would do anything for Miss Benjamin; in fact, she wished that there were some great deed she could perform just to show her love. Since there didn't seem to be, each day that she could find a flower or two, she faithfully took them to the loved teacher. When Mrs. Nelson, the good neighbor on the corner, gave her an entire bouquet for Miss Benjamin, the day was red-letter indeed.

About this time Mrs. Nelson seemed to feel that Helen needed something extra to brighten her life. She often watched the energetic little girl sprinting down the sidewalk to beat the "tardy bell."

"Helen," she called one day, "how would you like to have my June apple tree for your very own?"

The child was puzzled. "But I couldn't dig it up and take it home," she answered.

"Oh, no, I mean we'll leave it right where it is, but it will be your tree and you can eat the apples on it and be sure the tree is in good health," Mrs. Nelson replied with a smile.

"Oh, I'd love that!" Helen exclaimed. "Oh, thank you, Mrs. Nelson, thank you."

From then on, she inspected "her" tree several times a day. She stood at the bottom, peering into the branches, longing to climb it and explore the interesting little knobs of green near the top. But she couldn't make her legs start the upward climb. It was so high, so high.

School brought careful discipline from both parents. Father insisted that the three children must dress, wash, have breakfast, complete their assigned chores, and leave the kitchen in perfect order before they left.

"After all," he told them, "when you hear the first bell, all you have to do is run out the door and around the corner and there you are."

Mother added her instructions. "Under no circumstances are you ever to remain in the schoolyard after school is out," she told them firmly. "That is when children get into trouble.

You are to come home immediately."

There were other standards that must be met. Helen's parents insisted that they have every meal set on a tablecloth with cloth napkins. Both the tablecloths and napkins were made of a white "Indian head" material much used at that time. The material was so heavy that when the items had been sprinkled and left overnight, it took Helen hours of standing at the ironing board to iron them "properly"—that is, to Mother's satisfaction. From early childhood this was one of her tasks. If she hadn't gotten out all the wrinkles, or if the cloth had dried out too quickly, her mother would examine her work carefully, frown, hand the offending piece back to Helen and command, "Sprinkle it down and start over." The little girl, longing for the freedom of the outdoors, would go back to the ironing board with a lump in her throat.

Another tradition upheld fiercely in the Sanford home was that of a gracious Sunday dinner. After working six days, Mr. Sanford would, on Sunday morning, get out all the best linen and sterling silver and crystal he had inherited from his father. He and Helen would set the table perfectly on the gleaming cloth. They rolled the napkins, placing them in silver napkin rings. During the week he planned the meal and on Sunday he cooked it himself, giving his mother-in-law a day of rest. How Helen dreaded the cleaning up! There was an endless washing of dishes for her and her two brothers, who used every trick in the book to evade their part of the work and often succeeded, leaving her at the sink, hour after lonely hour. Those Sundays ended with her hands shriveled and pale from their long immersion in the hot, soapy dishwater. Of course Daddy often did the dishes and let her run out to play.

When Mr. Sanford felt that the family budget could bear the strain, he would take the three children for Sunday dinner to the Monarch Cafe on Virginia Street in Reno. The accoutrements were not nearly so gracious as those he insisted on at home, but Helen reveled in the prospect of a lovely afternoon—no cleaning up.

Christmases were awaited breathlessly, simple as they were. Each of the three children tried to save five dollars a year from the miniscule amounts of money they were given—a nickel here, a dime there. Then there was the joy of making out the shopping list. Just how much should be spent on each family member? Helen learned that if you spent twenty-five cents for Marvin, you should spend twenty-five cents for Harry, and maybe you really couldn't afford that much, because then there wouldn't be enough to spend on Mother and Daddy and Grandma and Dorothea—and new little cousin Janette, the apple of Helen's eye. How she envied Dorothea—a baby sister!

When mid-December came, the three of them walked to downtown Reno to the dime store, where they spent hours poring over their selections, figuring and refiguring their finances. The clerks knew them. They were welcome to stay as long as they liked. As for the tree, usually their father took them into the nearby mountains to select a wild evergreen. But these expeditions could turn into endurance contests, for he was by nature a dedicated perfectionist in everything he did. The tree must be perfect. If, after hours of looking in the cold wind, a totally perfect one could not be found, when they arrived home with the tree they had selected Mr. Sanford would drill holes in the trunk and carefully insert the extra branches he had cut from other trees so that the tree presented a picture of symmetrical beauty.

The tree was then decorated carefully with the few simple ornaments the family owned and the gifts wrapped neatly—Helen learned to wrap packages like a professional as soon as she could read—and piled around it. On Christmas morning the children were not allowed into the room with the tree until they had eaten breakfast and had gone through the usual routine of cleaning up. They could not come to the table without having their hair perfectly brushed and their clothes in good order.

"I will not have frowzy children in this house," their father said firmly. "Christmas is no exception."

And so the days came and went. Helen grew up with a sense of little self-worth. Her mother was by nature undemonstrative, though Helen sensed dimly that had she been able to do so, she would have verbalized the love that was in her heart. Her warm father, Helen's idol, never realized the damage he did to his lonely little daughter by his "left-handed compliments." He was a great tease. When Helen would have a new dress, a rare happening, he might say tenderly, "Why, isn't she just the ugliest little thing?" The little girl, literal and uncomprehending, heard the words, not the loving tone. The conviction grew in her small heart that she was unattractive. She would always be unattractive. She must work harder than anyone else and make herself as useful as possible to make up for this. She could not know that she was a beautiful little girl with large, luminous blue eyes that mirrored all her thoughts. As the years passed, and her height was the subject of family mirth, she had no way of realizing that she was tall, willowy, and lovely; she was Helen, the "beanpole."

Helen felt like a failure on one specific account. Her mother told her teasingly, "I married your father so my children would have his beautiful, red, curly hair. And you don't have it. You just have light-brown hair. Why didn't you have red hair?"

The child could not understand the humor. She knew only that she had failed. Before her mother became ill, each day she had curled Helen's hair into ringlets that framed her square little face glowingly. But the sickness changed all that. Hurriedly now, each morning Grandmother braided her soft light-brown hair so tightly that the little girl felt she could hardly blink her eyes. Later, when "Dutch bobs" became popular, Helen begged for one. "Never!" her mother told her. "With your square face it would be a disaster!" Once Helen tearfully cut a few strands above her forehead, lost her courage, and hid the strands behind her dresser. As she grew she sometimes seemed like a young colt, with arms and legs too long for her body. She was used to being told impatiently, "Helen, it's impossible to find clothes to fit your arms and legs!" Another failure. Even had slacks been heard of then, Etta Sanford would not have permitted Helen to wear them. They "pertained to a man."

Harry and Marvin were very protective of their little sister, though they teased her unmercifully, often making her life a burden to her. One day Harry came into his mother's room and remarked emphatically, "I hope you won't let Helen go around half-dressed like some of the girls." It turned out that on his way home he'd seen some girls playing on the jungle gym who were hanging upside down, and their scanty undergarments had revealed much more of their anatomy than he considered proper. He needn't have worried about Helen. Her mother and grandmother saw to it that she wore black bloomers to school, with strict instructions to keep the elastic just above her knees. On Sabbath, as the years went on, she had a pair of white bloomers—but with the same modest cut.

Promptness was another Sanford tenet. You simply were never late for anything—for church, for school, for a social engagement. And you had to allow enough time to leave the house in good order and still be prompt for your appointments. Probably this insistence produced a considerable degree of tension in a household that was, to some extent, motherless and that contained an invalid who must be cared for.

Helen's silent, inner fears continued and grew. When she was "farmed out" to baby sitters from time to time, she was afraid—afraid of doing something wrong. When she was about 6, her mother arranged for her to have piano lessons on their old square piano. She hated those times for she was deathly afraid of the picture hanging above the instrument. The stern, forbidding, bearded visage was considered to be one of the family ancestors—a judge. Did pictures ever come down out of their frames? Helen was afraid to ask. But oh, the joy when for no announced reason her mother decreed that this picture should be removed and a print of a lovely English garden substituted. But that was not the only fear. When her fingers—long for her age—stumbled on the keys, her teacher struck them sharply with a ruler. It was not just the stinging pain she dreaded. It was the renewed sense of insecurity, of being so worthless that she must be punished.

Ben Sanford idolized his wife. Her bright, blithe spirit, so stimulating, so intoxicating, was dimmed by her illness, but it remained as real to him as when he had first met her. She was always more wife than mother; their relationship was romantic, close. In her personal grooming she was fastidious and meticulous. With iron determination and superhuman effort, all through her long illness she kept her hair neat and her bedwear becoming, and on the rare occasions when she felt well enough to be up and with the family, she was dressed carefully and beautifully.

Ben was absolutely determined that Etta would live. With his gallantry, he fostered her feeling that she was loved, admired, cherished. He gave her a reason to live, to keep on fighting. And for herself, she was no quitter. Each spring, when the florist got his first shipment of spring flowers, tight as the family budget was, Ben brought her a bunch of violets in the very special green tissue wrapping that florists use. When the autumn came, he brought her a big chrysanthemum, which she always put in a large brown vase. The flower could be counted on to last a week. And he was always on a tireless search for new foods that would tempt her scanty appetite. His loving devotion to his wife became almost a legend in the city of Reno.

Helen's concepts of marriage relationships were formed by her father's actions. She would always measure other men in her life by that yardstick.

But the dark threads of unhappiness in the home never

abated. The three children talked endlessly and fearfully of what they would do if their mother died. When Mother's fever climbed, her cheeks flushed and her eyes dulled, the bedroom was off-limits to them. But sick as she was, she represented security, especially to Helen. Would anyone else love a little girl with just plain brown hair and long arms and legs? Unsure as she sometimes was of her mother's love, her terror was a palpable thing as she contemplated life without the crisp, firm presence of Etta Sanford.

Another of Helen's sadnesses concerned the Parent-Teacher Association meetings. The teachers made large charts with the names of every child in the room. When a parent attended the meeting, a large star was placed beside the name. With Helen, the hurt went deep when there was never a star for her. When her teachers, unthinking, scolded the child because she couldn't produce a parent, the little girl mumbled red-faced apologies. With an invalid mother, an overworked father, and a tired-out grandmother, there simply was not enough of anything to go around.

As the years progressed Ben Sanford and his little girl were embarrassed because their house was becoming very run-down. There was not a cent to spend for paint or for repairs. If a repair did not require money, Ben took care of it. Otherwise, financial stringency precluded it. But the inside of the home was always spotless. He found leftover pieces of linoleum that matched the kitchen floor, and each time a spot in the kitchen wore out, he would carefully cut and fit a piece to match perfectly.

An incident during this period made an indelible impression on Helen's mind. Her aunt and uncle from Sacramento, wealthy society people, made a visit in the midst of the hot Reno summer. Aware as they were of the almost-desperate financial plight of the family, they had never offered any kind of help. On this visit, they continued aloof from the desperate need of the family, with one exception. Childless themselves, they offered to adopt Helen.

"Just think what we could do for her," Ben's sister-in-law urged, glancing disdainfully about the shabby bedroom where the conversation was carried on. Turning to Etta, she remarked unfeelingly, "You certainly aren't able to do anything for her yourself."

Her eyes wide with shock and outrage, Etta gasped, "You mean you would try to take my little girl away from me just because I'm sick?"

Overhearing it all, Helen was caught between fear that her parents might give her away, and a deep, warm joy that her mother loved her enough to keep her. And when, from time to time, her mother gave her pretty little pieces of her own jewelry, such as a sapphire ring and a bracelet, her delight in wearing them was doubled because her mother had given them to her.

Helen had done so well at the beginning of first grade that she was promoted to the second, which she mastered with equal ease, except for math, which continued to be a lifelong bugaboo. On grade-card day, she couldn't wait to rush home with her grade card, which she showed first to her mother, then to Mrs. Nelson, the June apple-tree giver, and then her father, when he returned home from work. Probably Helen's rapid scholastic progress was, to some extent, the result of her mother's avid reading habits. The latter was never without a book, and the three children picked up her love of reading. Helen was always going to the public library, checking out as many books as she was allowed, taking them home and reading them almost overnight, and then going back for more. However, if a book was sad, such as *Pollyanna,* she cried so hard that Etta had to take the book from her.

Etta also believed in thrift. As the children grew older, she gave each of them little black metal banks that could be opened only at the bank downtown. She encouraged the three to save every penny they possibly could; from time to time, when the banks actually became full, they were taken downtown and deposited in the accounts she had opened for them. A dollar saved was a large amount of money.

Though Etta Sanford's nature was not very demonstrative toward her children, she had a quick and total empathy for the handicapped or those afflicted with physical problems. Nothing could arouse her formidable anger more than an unsympathetic remark about someone less fortunate. Helen's own growing compassion for those in trouble stemmed from her mother's influence.

"We are here on this earth to do all we can to help people who need help," her mother said.

As the days and years flew by, another indelible impression was being etched on Helen's receptive mind—that of the unswerving devotion of one marriage partner to another, the faithfulness through crippling illness, the absence of complaining. When people married, if one person became sick and helpless, the well person took care of the sick one. She had only to look at her father to know that.

CHAPTER 3

Living and Learning

BUT Etta's illness got no better. It dominated the family's life. Tossing in her bed, only her strength of character and iron determination kept her from adding her despair to her husband's already crushing burdens. Each time a new doctor set up practice in Reno, Ben Sanford arranged as soon as possible for him to examine Etta, hoping that perhaps some new method of treatment might be suggested. But the search seemed hopeless. She grew weaker and thinner month by month. Now there were large tubercular abscesses under her arms; there was pus around her fingernails and under her toenails. For this fastidious, high-spirited woman, the humiliation of feeling that she was an object of repugnance added to her anguish.

It seemed only a matter of time.

By now Harry, Marvin, and Helen had been attending Sabbath school rather regularly, and Etta Sanford seemed to consider herself a Seventh-day Adventist, the rebellious philosophical storms now a thing of the past. During the long hours of her illness, when she was too sick to read or to embroider or mend, she tossed on her bed as the kaleidoscope of thoughts raced through her weary mind. The old familiar teachings of her young girlhood came back with crystal clarity; there had been such a note of certainty to it. God was real. He had given His Son. He had given truth to this small body of people.

"Mother, I think you would enjoy prayer meeting at the Adventist church," Etta said one day, startling her mother considerably, more to humor the invalid than anything else. Her mother agreed to attend, did so, and found the small handful of believers a great comfort and reinforcement. Gradually, the Sanford family began to regard themselves as at least "semi"-Adventists. They kept up, to some extent, with what was going on in the little church and the larger body it represented.

Helen responded to Sabbath school with the enthusiasm that was so much a part of her nature. When the classes formed in the children's division, after the opening songs and the prayer and the mission story, the teacher took out the class record and asked very seriously, "Now who studied the lesson seven times this past week?"

Little Helen never studied seven times; no one took an interest in seeing that she did so. But the other class members were so hostile to anyone who broke the perfect record that she fell into the habit of whispering "Seven" when the teacher glanced her way. Being rejected by the class members was a fate she couldn't face. As a matter of fact, the other children never invited her to their homes or included her in any activities, just as the adult members did not include the Sanford family. All through her growing years, this was a heartache to Helen. (At her own wedding, in the same church, the mystery was solved when one of the members said to her, "Helen, I never dreamed you'd marry a preacher. None of us wanted our children to play with you because your Aunt Clara was not a Seventh-day Adventist.")

The church school teacher was Helen's Sabbath school teacher. She was one of the main reasons the little girl attended so faithfully. Helen loved the pretty silk dresses the young teacher wore, and fantasized as to how the silk would feel if ever she had the courage to touch one little segment of it. Also, with the Sabbath school class held in the church school room, Helen enjoyed looking at the assignments on the board, which she found easy to read. The handwriting of the teacher was an object of beauty to her, for she loved beauty intensely.

One song that Helen especially loved was "A Child of the

King." With the great depression permeating every aspect of her life, it was thrilling to think of a God who was rich in "houses and lands" as well as "rubies and diamonds." Lustily she sang, " 'His coffers are full—He has riches untold,' " not having the slightest idea of what a coffer might be. It was an exhilarating experience for her to declare in song that " 'I'm a child of the King, a child of the King! With Jesus, my Saviour, I'm a child of the King!' "

Another stanza popular during depression days was the following:

A tent or a cottage, O why should I care?
They're building a palace for me over there!
Though exiled from home, yet still I may sing:
"All glory to God, I'm a child of the King."

Small Helen, with her shining blue eyes, her intrepid spirit, her rich imagination, could not even imagine that years later, almost a bride, she would stand beside a handsome someone and sing this same stanza—and end up living with her someone in the aforementioned tent!

Although the church members themselves seemed unable or unwilling to meet the needs of the Sanford family, the conference president and his wife felt differently. At that time the office of the Nevada-Utah Conference was situated in Reno. Elder and Mrs. M. L. Rice heard of the Sanfords, called on them, and a strong friendship grew up between Etta Sanford and Mrs. Rice; the latter found Etta's sparkling wit and incisive logic stimulating. The church members were not entirely pleased with this development; mutters were heard that the Sanfords were monopolizing Elder and Mrs. Rice. But Mrs. Rice's beautiful sympathy, expressed so lovingly, and her very real concern for the three children, especially little Helen, were like rain on the parched desert to the Sanfords.

One summer day, Etta Sanford called her mother to her bed. "Please phone Elder Rice and ask him if he will take me to camp meeting," she directed, as though her request were the most natural and ordinary in the world.

Stupefied, her mother gasped, "You'll die if you undertake that kind of trip!"

Etta replied, "Well, I'm already dying. I know it; you know it; Ben knows it; every doctor in Reno knows it. If I'm going to die, I'd just as soon die going to camp meeting. Now go down into the basement in the storage closet and bring up a dress for me to wear."

There was no arguing with Etta when she was in this mood. Her mother phoned Elder and Mrs. Rice; they talked over the request and then decided that Etta had a right to take her destiny into her own hands, since she was, as she said, dying. They would take her to camp meeting for a day. Then her mother rummaged in the basement for a dress, the smallest she could find of her daughter's wardrobe. When Etta stood to her feet, shakily, and tried on the dress, it hung grotesquely on her emaciated form.

"Well, nobody cares what I look like," she declared spiritedly. "I'll comb my hair as nicely as I can and have everything very neat, and that will have to do."

Elder and Mrs. Rice still had a few reservations about the plan. "Now you must tell us when you have had all your strength will take," they made her promise.

As the car sped along—and it was a rare treat to Etta, for the Sanfords could not afford a car—she enjoyed the outdoors with the intensity that only one who expects soon to leave the world can feel. Camp meeting was held in a lovely apple orchard west of Reno, along the Truckee River. Chism's Orchard even had a well with a wooden bucket and irrigation ditches running through the grove where people put watermelons and other foods to keep them ice-cold. The ditches were fed by water running down directly from the High Sierra Mountains surrounding Reno.

That first day Etta lasted through only one meeting. Almost dazed with fatigue, she asked to be taken home, where her mother had to put her to bed as one would take care of a child. But she was determined to return the next day. Nothing could shake her resolution. "If I'm going to die, it might as well be at camp meeting," she told her husband again.

Helen, hearing this, crept off by herself. If only Mother weren't sick—the refrain beat endlessly in her mind. When I'm grown up and married, nobody is ever going to be sick in my house. And nobody is going to be afraid.

By the end of camp meeting, Etta was staying for the entire day of meetings. When a call was made for those who wished to take their stand and join the church, she was the first to raise her hand.

"But how in the world can you be baptized outdoors in that cold Truckee River?" Ben asked her, aghast.

"Just the way everyone else is," she told him.

She went forward in faith, feeling that in her doomed condition there was little to live for and that whatever happened was all right. She realized that rebaptism was a necessary step for her to take in starting a new life style.

God rewarded her faith and courage. From that time forward the active tuberculosis disappeared. God did not restore her crooked back or her damaged lung, but never again did she have a positive test for tuberculosis. She was very, very weak; she would never be as strong as before; but the imminent danger of death had been taken away. As the years went on, she was more and more able to keep her home, do a bit of yardwork, and even walk a mile to town.

The family was not immediately aware of the great load that had been lifted from their hearts. The realization came gradually. For Helen, though, another bereavement followed close on the heels of her mother's baptism. Her grandmother had been, next to her father, the most stable factor in her life. She loved the tiny, short, plump little lady with all the pent-up affection of her warm heart. Her love was returned unreservedly; Helen's grandmother, weary though she was with the never-ending work, saw to it that she and

Helen had a few "fun times" together in the midst of whatever she was doing. When Helen was 8, Ben Sanford decided that her grandmother simply must have a rest. "Mother," he told her, "I want you to take a trip back to upstate New York and visit all your relatives."

Stunned, she stammered, "Why, I couldn't possibly—why, you need me here. How will you manage?"

"Don't you worry," he assured her. "We'll hire someone to come in and help. Helen's a big girl now and the boys are strong and I want you to have the time of your life."

Money was gotten together somehow for the train ticket, and before Helen knew it, Grandma was gone. Would she ever come back? Lonely now, the little girl wondered and wondered. After six months, when another train brought her home again, it was a happy day.

Perhaps because of her even more acute loneliness now, Helen began to think of God in a very personal way. The lessons she heard at Sabbath school translated themselves into beautiful realities. There was a God in heaven who loved her. He would always be with her. Perhaps Mother might die, and Grandmother might go away, and Father might have to spend all his time at the store, but God would always stay close to her.

One time, outdoors in the warm Reno night, she saw the sliver of a new moon in the sky. Running inside, she exclaimed to her father, "Daddy, the moon looks just like God's fingernail!"

But she was a totally normal little girl, full of mischief, full of plans and activities, the latter quality now making her popular at school. Eager for a bit of money all her own, she approached the local grocery store, run by Mr. and Mrs. Wiggs. The Sanford children went to the store several times a day, as did most people of that era. Since the Sanfords possessed only an old ice chest for refrigeration, perishable food had to be purchased largely from meal to meal.

"Mrs. Wiggs," Helen suggested one day, "if I make

potholders, will you sell them here in your store for me?"

Impressed by the ingenuity of the little girl, Mrs. Wiggs agreed that she would sell any potholders Helen produced, at the price of two for a quarter. And so Helen added another activity to her list.

With no girls in the neighborhood except her cousin Dorothea and her little sister, Helen played with the groups of boys who flocked around the Sanford home, friends of Harry and Marvin. She learned to be totally at ease with boys, learned to accept their teasing (though not always gracefully) and often to outdistance and outperform them in their own games.

Now a new anxiety appeared. Both Ben and Etta Sanford gave thanks each day for the cessation of her tuberculosis. But as time passed, it was obvious that the disease had seriously injured her spine. Her leg was becoming numb so rapidly that local physicians told her it would be only a matter of time until she would be helpless. She must have spinal surgery. A dear friend in San Francisco insisted that she come to her, that the surgery could be done much more safely in the more sophisticated hospitals of San Francisco.

"I'm reluctant to accept room and board and so much care from Lois," she told her mother, now back from the East.

"I believe that she really wants to do this for you. So I'll take you to San Francisco on the train, then come back and take care of the house and children while you have the surgery," her mother told her.

When the two of them left, Helen waved and waved until the train was out of sight into the mountains. Her father said nothing, but she noticed tears in his eyes and the strain on his face, though as a child she had no vocabulary for that word. Only as an adult did she realize that he must have wondered whether he would ever see his wife, his sweetheart, again. Surgery was then very risky—and he could not give her even the reassurance of his presence, for he must keep food on the table for the children and a roof over their heads.

After Etta had been examined by the physician most qualified for the surgery and he assured her that it could be done, she was stunned to find that the price would be $2,000.

"Two thousand dollars!" she exclaimed to her friend Lois on the way home. "It might as well be 2 million! I'm going to pack tonight and call Mother to come and take me back to Reno."

"No, you're not," Lois told her. "We're not finished yet. I'm going to take you over to the clinic at the University of California. They do things for people who haven't the funds to pay."

Not wanting to offend her friend, Etta agreed. The two women filled out the forms, made the application—and, to their amazement, saw the same doctor, who, in his private office, had told them that the price would be $2,000. Now it would be, for the most part, free. Proud as she was, Etta knew she must accept this help for the sake of her children and Ben. In June, 1925, she had a spinal fusion of four vertebrae, and had to remain there, first in the hospital and then with her friend Lois, until Thanksgiving.

She missed her family greatly, small Helen in particular. Lying in bed, her back aching, she would visualize the eager, smiling face, the large, shining blue eyes, the soft brown hair, the skinned knees, the rough little hands. A lump would come to her throat, and over and over she would pray, "Dear Lord, please take care of Helen for me. Please do for her what I cannot do. Keep her safe."

Hating to be idle, she began helping Lois make elegant handkerchiefs from voile and linen, with intricate embroidered designs and the most delicate of hand-rolled hems. Then, after returning to Reno, she sold more than four hundred of these beautiful handkerchiefs for one dollar each, a very large price indeed for that day and age.

As the years went on and Etta's health improved, she

constantly made aprons and other items to sell. Her hands were never idle, especially during the long months and years she was in bed. After the children were married and on their own, she used her needlework skills to provide money for Sabbath school Investment, sent small sums to a former church school teacher who was studying medicine, helped to educate a little Indian child, and gave little gifts to nearly everyone who came to visit. A padded coat hanger, a pretty handkerchief—she loved to give these simple things, which represented the simple yet warm Sanford life style.

Her mother's long absence created an ache in Helen's small heart that in time she accepted as normal. Painstakingly she composed letters, writing them with extreme neatness, knowing her mother's high standards of excellence. "I miss you," she wrote week after week. But Grandmother's warm presence was a solid rock of reassurance. Then one day a phone call came. They had thought Mother could not return until Christmas, and now she was telling them that her progress had been such that she could come at Thanksgiving.

"If Mother will come and get me, I can come home," she told them joyfully.

During the few days of waiting, Helen was consumed with a new worry. She was afraid that she didn't even remember what her mother looked like. Would she recognize her when she got off the train? Then a new thought struck even more terror. Suppose her mother didn't recognize *her!* It had been so long.

But then the day came. Helen was afraid to go to the station with the family. But if she told them that, they would laugh at her, and they might even think she didn't want to see her mother! Paralyzed by the dilemma, she crawled into a closet and hid in the dark for a while. Daddy had been so busy, and Grandmother so busy, and there really wasn't much place for a little girl. Probably they wouldn't even miss her if she stayed by herself. But when she heard Daddy calling sharply, "Helen!" she scurried out, and walked down the street, her heart almost suffocating her, it beat so hard.

Then the train pulled into the station with much puffing and smoking. The baggage man walked to the doors of the baggage car, opened them, and he and her father and others helped lift her mother down on her stretcher, her grandmother beside her. And instantly Helen recognized that loved face which changed to a glow of brightness when the little girl hurled herself upon the stretcher, her arms wide. Ben had ordered an ambulance to take Etta to the house; then there was the joyful reunion. And all too soon, the familiar words, "Now we must let Mother rest."

The winter set in, cold and bitter as it often was in Reno, so close to the High Sierras. Grandma and two young uncles now made their home with the Sanfords. Since the house was too small to accommodate all of them, the three children slept on the porch, even in the dead of winter. The howling wind would swirl the snow in onto their beds. Going to bed each night was an endurance contest; it would have been unendurable had not the children learned to heat the big flatirons, wrap them in newspaper, pin outing flannel around them, and put them in the beds some time before they retired.

One dark, cold February morning about five o'clock, Helen's father came out onto the porch in the bitter cold and shook the three children awake. With a sob in his voice, he told them, "Grandmother is dead."

Dazed, uncomprehending, shivery, Helen was too stunned to cry. How could Grandmother be dead? She had gotten sick about a week ago, and they said she had a ruptured appendix; but to the child that meant nothing. She fled to her mother's room, but the latter's low sobbing struck further terror to her heart. The fear and insecurity rushed over her in a frightening wave. Grandmother could not leave her. She needed Grandmother; she had to have her.

Though she was taken to the funeral home to see her

grandmother, the still form in the casket bore little resemblance to the lively, spirited, energetic little lady who had been the solace of her life. Helen sat through the funeral numb with shock, and at the cemetery afterward she listlessly followed her parents from the grave, the cold wind whipping around her legs.

"I don't think Grandmother is really gone!" she burst out when the family had made the sad journey home. "I'm not going to believe it."

Her parents exchanged glances over her head.

"But you must believe it, Helen," her mother told her quietly. "We cannot bring her back. We can only remember how much we loved her and never forget her."

Silent, the child was not convinced. For months, though she said nothing to anyone else, she went out to the sidewalk many times a day and glanced up and down, hoping, hoping that Grandma would be coming home. Each day she told herself that Grandma would come the next day. "Grandma would never leave me," Helen whispered to herself. "She loves me."

The death of her grandmother was not only a keen heartache for the family; it presented Ben Sanford with another crisis. The surgeon had told Etta that she must not do any real work for at least two years if she expected a full recovery from her serious spinal surgery. When Ben found her in the kitchen lifting some cans from one location to another, he was horrified.

"Stop that!" he told her. "You know better than that."

She smiled wryly. "Ben, you made a poor bargain when you married me. I've been nothing but trouble for you—and someone has to step in here and do some of the work. I've been in that bed for so many years; it's certainly my turn."

He put his arms around her. "Don't you ever say I made a poor bargain," he told her tenderly. "And I'm going to get some household help."

"How will we pay for it?" she whispered fearfully.

"I'll worry about that," he told her.

He did get help, in the person of Lena Serafina Wilbur, a little German lady, who did some of the cooking. But there was always so much work to be done that Etta could not restrain herself. Her back never healed properly.

Though Helen's childhood had been more full of work than that of many other little girls, Ben and Etta had seen to it that there was time for flying about the sidewalks on her bicycle and on her skates, with her long, long legs pumping up and down furiously. She had always been an active child, almost compulsively needing exercise and fresh air.

Once in later years, Etta said to Helen philosophically, "You know, it's probably just as well that my back healed crookedly, for if it had healed as straight and stiff as it was supposed to, I would never in the world have been able to get my shoes and stockings on by myself. Imagine if I had had to have someone help me do that every day!"

Helen, more caught up now in school life, was five feet eight inches tall by the time she was 13—a condition her brothers never let her forget, even when, during the daily after-school ball games, she led the cheerleading section in their behalf. In junior high, she was put into the "A" section, composed of superior students, which meant that she was loaded down with such amounts of homework each night that she wondered whether the honor of being thought of as bright was worth the penalty. Her growing interest in art, a subject she had loved since earliest childhood, now began to blossom. When the seventh-grade girls were given six weeks of cooking, then sewing, then art, to identify the interest they might like to pursue as electives, there was no doubt in Helen's mind as to her preference. Ever since first grade all her teachers had said to Helen, "You have a real gift in art." Now a golden moment came.

"Helen, your work shows such promise that we want to place you in the advanced art class," the principal told her.

In the midst of her delight, suddenly a worm of anxiety

wriggled into her mind. Helen remembered having heard other students mention that although everything in the public school was supplied to the students in most cases, with the depression now in full swing, students in the advanced art class had to buy paints and art paper and brushes and certain books and other supplies. Her spirits dropped like a thud as swiftly as they had soared.

"I don't want to join that class," she mumbled to the principal, red-faced, miserable, her pride forbidding her to make a clean breast of the problem.

"But Helen—you're so talented! You're the most talented student in art in the seventh grade. I thought you'd be so happy!"

Knowing that she seemed ungrateful and boorish, still Helen could think of no other way out of her predicament than the one she had chosen. She continued to insist that she didn't want to take the class, wasn't interested, and wouldn't do it.

On the way home, she blinked back tears. She would have loved the art class more than anything else in the world. But I could never ask Daddy for that money, she thought to herself. We can just barely scrape by financially as it is.

The principal, sensing that a deeper problem lay beneath the surface, called Helen's father. "Can't you persuade her to take the art class?" she requested.

Her father met with no better luck and, all unsuspecting, he told the principal, "Well, if she doesn't want to take the class, I'm not willing to force her to take it."

In later life, Helen bitterly regretted her decision. Her father probably would have found the money, which was really not a large amount, but which to Helen's young eyes had seemed a fortune.

Her consciousness of the value of money had been sharpened by the hone of need. In addition to the potholders she had continued to make and sell, she grew maiden-hair ferns. Since these delicate ferns were not native to the arid

State of Nevada, Helen felt fortunate that some elderly ladies whom her parents had befriended gave her small cuttings. These she carefully nourished and tended until they became plants large enough to sell. By the time she was 11 or 12 she had learned that at the Sunday ball games, refreshments were popular. She began baking cakes in the old coal-burning stove, learning to gauge the temperature and to keep it constant so that her cakes wouldn't fall. An especially popular cake was her spice with butter frosting. Her brothers and their friends paid for these cakes in "cold cash." In fact, they were much less serious about money than Helen, running out of money frequently before they got paid, though now they were all steadily employed. When they asked to borrow a dollar from Helen, she made the stipulation that if they borrowed one dollar on Friday, they owed her *two* dollars on Saturday and if they waited for repayment until Sunday they owed *three* dollars! Her brothers still remind her frequently of her "extortion."

By this time—and long before, actually—Helen was ironing at least fifteen shirts each week. The boys were home, and so were the two young uncles who had taken up residence with the family. After the shirts came back from the wet wash, starch had to be cooked on the stove and strained to remove lumps; then the shirts were dipped in the mess. The band of the shirts with detachable collars had to be starched exactly right or the collar button wouldn't fit properly. But if you got that immensely thick starch on the body of the shirt itself, you had to start over, rinsing the shirt and wringing it out and restarching. With no automatic irons, it was a feat of skill not to scorch the shirts. Also, the irons had to be scraped frequently to remove the brown accumulated starch.

Junior high was more than a mile away, with no cafeteria. Most of the children who lived at such a distance brought their lunch, but not the Sanford children. They raced home (the lunch period lasted for an hour and a quarter) and Helen fixed the lunch, then cleaned up the kitchen, knowing that if she did not do this she would have it to do after school.

The association between Helen and her brothers and young uncles was close and warm. As she became taller and more mature, her mother often looked at her a bit speculatively when she would perch on the laps of one of the boys. One day she called her into the bedroom.

"Helen," she said gently, "you really are getting to be a big girl now. I don't want you to sit on the boys' laps anymore."

That was all she said. But Helen understood and subsequently developed the necessary reserve in her contacts.

And so the days and months passed, with quilting, with Helen's "ditch garden" down by the retaining wall around the irrigation ditch, and with the rigid routine and high standards of her home. In summer, during hot afternoons, she sat and embroidered or crocheted, a skill she had mastered. At times the family sat together while one of them read the Bible aloud and, beg as they might, their mother never permitted the children to skip over the hard words. They did the best they could.

But times worsened as the depression became deeper. Now the Sanfords could no longer afford to send the laundry to the wet wash. "Helen," her father told her, "you are going to have to do the washing for the family. I know it's a lot to ask. But Mother cannot do it, and someone must."

The child—for she was still a child, tall though she was—gulped. Again she must manage, one way or another. Her father fixed a washboard that fitted across the bathtub, and Helen bent over it all day long Sundays, washing, rinsing, and wringing. It became routine for her to go to school on Monday mornings with her hands so blistered from wringing sheets and shirts that she could hardly bear the touch of a pencil.

The yearly housecleaning was a family enterprise that

took place during the time when the teachers attended the teachers' institutes in the autumn. Helen and Marvin and Harry would go through one room at a time, while their frail mother sat in a rocking chair, watching them with eagle eyes. In the bedrooms, every dresser drawer had to be emptied out and rearranged. The drawers had to be scrubbed inside and out. The backs of the dressers were wiped down and the door frames and walls and ceilings scrubbed. The young folks took the rugs out on the line and beat them. To lessen the drudgery their mother read to the three children as they moved through the house, room by room. Never having known any other kind of life, Helen assumed that all people worked as hard as they and bore their share of family responsibilities.

Sometimes the spirited, energetic teen-ager would long wistfully for pretty clothes and for something else—what, she did not specifically know. She was going through the uncertainties and unhappiness of the early teen, but she had little time to dwell on her own problems. The United States was locked into the depression; night and day haggard men came to the door, begging for food, only their great need compelling them to this ultimate humiliation. Her mother and dad fed them all, out of the slender larder of the family, usually asking them to take on some small task so as to preserve their self-respect.

CHAPTER 4
A New Life Direction

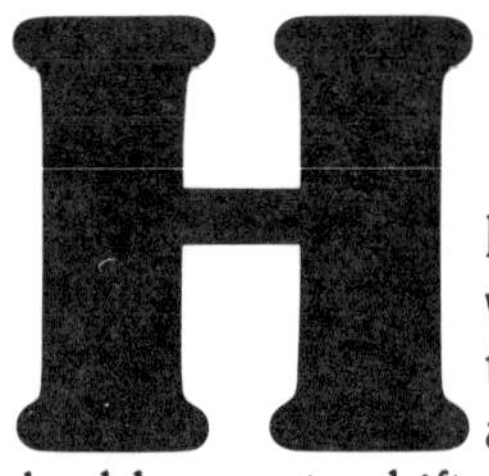

HELEN had continued to feel that God was a presence in her life, but in spite of the healing her mother had experienced and her baptism, somehow the family had begun to drift away from the Adventist Church. From time to time they attended the Lutheran church, partly because of the frequent visits of the Lutheran pastor and partly because of the social life, so long absent from the lives of the Sanford family. The beautiful, warm suppers held in the church basement by the Lutherans were a great drawing card.

One Sabbath afternoon as the family sat on the screened porch, rocking in the hot stillness, one of the Adventist members came up the walk. "There are going to be some meetings I think you people would be interested in," he told them, and gave Helen's mother a handbill. She looked down at it and saw that Elder Phillip Knox, a totally new name to her, would hold meetings in a nearby auditorium. He was advertised as an astronomer who would show many pictures.

Suddenly she made up her mind. "Let's plan to attend these meetings," she told her family. "I think we might enjoy them—and anyway, the meetings are free and it's something to do besides going to all those evening ball games. Maybe all of you will stop eating so many hot dogs and mustard!"

The Sanford family was there on opening night. They loved the sermon. They enjoyed the pictures. Helen was literally transported by the music; it seemed to her that she had been searching for this special feeling all through her short life. Phillip Knox was a man of unlimited energy and enthusiasm. At one point he invited all those interested to meet him in the schoolyard at two in the morning to view the stars. Helen set an alarm clock, dressed herself, and, shivering in the night air, was a delighted participant, scanning the heavens.

"Oh, all this is so interesting!" she assured her parents over and over. "We're studying ancient history in school right now, and it's so wonderful to hear Pastor Knox interpret all these things in the light of prophecy."

Imperceptibly Helen's heart was flooded with the joy of fellowship with Christ. Each morning was a joy when, on awakening, she realized that she could ask Christ to walk with her through the long days of study and work. He would be with her. She need not feel alone and insecure. She wanted the whole world to know of this joy that had come into her life.

"Mother, I want to be baptized," she announced.

Her mother was ambivalent. "Are you sure that you understand all that is involved in being baptized into the Adventist Church, Helen?" she asked. "I think you had better talk with Elder Knox."

It was arranged that the conversation would take place on the screened porch. Helen, only 13, awkward and unsure of herself, could hardly remember the conversation. She did know, however, that she truly wanted to be baptized. Realizing her sincerity, Elder Knox agreed that she should take the step.

Finding a baptismal site for the candidates was a problem in Reno. Finally it was decided that Bower's Springs would be rented—a popular hot springs where the young people of the town loved to go when they could afford the fifty cents' admission fee. For the Sanford children, it was the treat of their lives if they could afford one swim per summer. Helen couldn't swim, having had so little opportunity to learn, but she loved the water. She and another girl who was also being baptized talked it over with the logic of childhood.

"Isn't it a shame to waste all that wonderful water?" they

asked each other. "Let's wear our bathing suits under our baptismal robes and swim for a while afterward!"

Helen's mother, overhearing the conversation, didn't know whether to scold or smile. Gently she pointed out the inappropriateness of the idea. And when the day came, swimming was the furthest thing from Helen's thoughts. The solemnity of the baptism, the call to discipleship, sounded so strongly in her ears that she was deaf to the sights and sounds around her. She arose from the water truly to walk in "newness of life," a resolve that would never waver. Ben Sanford and Marvin were baptized with her. It was a new beginning.

Helen's baptism marked an enormous change and turning point. Until now, she had loved the movies and lived for the new ones that came to the theaters, treating herself as often as she felt she could spare the fifteen or twenty cents' admission fee. Now she did not go.

"Mother," she said, "I want to follow Christ all the way. I'm not going to wear my jewelry anymore."

Her mother, knowing how the tall, blue-eyed girl loved her many necklaces and rings and bracelets, felt a momentary pang. "You must do what you think is right, Helen," she told her.

But it was a struggle. When her grandmother had died, she had left Helen some of her pretty jewelry. Helen was so used to wearing it with her plain dresses that she felt almost naked and unclothed without it. She struggled against the disappointment she felt, the sorrow it caused her not to wear the beautiful baubles. Sturdily she said to herself, "I can wear all of these things in heaven. Jesus is asking me to give them up just for a little while so that I won't become vain and forget that without Him I am nothing. Surely I can do this much for Him."

Ben Sanford had also found the meetings an answer to many of the longings and questions in his heart. He too had felt the great desire for commitment by baptism. But there were his cigarettes. He would not risk being baptized and then bring reproach on the church by becoming a hypocrite.

"I am going to put myself to the test," he told his family. "I am going to keep a full pack of cigarettes in the cash register for two weeks, and if I can manage not to smoke even one, then I think I can safely be baptized." He too would never subsequently waver.

Then a stunning blow fell. Since he could no longer work at the meat market on Saturday, he was fired.

"What will we do? How will we get along?" Etta Sanford asked fearfully. Helen silently echoed the questions. Must life always be this way? Must there always be fear and insecurity and sickness and poverty?

"The Lord will take care of us if we do the very best we can," Ben Sanford insisted stoutly. And they did manage to scrape by, just barely, though their lives narrowed further and further as the weeks and months passed, and he worked at an unfamiliar salesman's job in Reno and the surrounding area. He always managed to sell just barely enough dry goods to keep the family in food and under a roof.

But they were happy in the newfound love of God. Their lives were so changed they often wondered if they were the same Sanford family. Instead of pork and sausage and coffee, they had clean meat and fruits and vegetables. Helen, determined to live up to every suggestion, every nuance that came her way, caused herself a great deal of heartache, taking much of the joy out of her young life, joy that was hers by right.

"You know," she said to her parents, "some of the ladies at the church think it is wrong to have bobbed hair, so I'm going to let my hair grow out."

Her mother was startled. "What will you do with it, Helen?" she asked gently.

"Why, I'll wear it in a knot on the back of my neck," Helen declared.

Her mother remonstrated gently. "But your hair is so

thick and wiry—do you think you can manage it?"

"I'll have to," Helen retorted grimly. In due time she was the owner of a little knot of wiry hair on her neck, so stubborn and unruly that at times, as she would sit studying, there would be a little *ping*, and a hairpin would jump from the knot and land across the room. This hairstyle gave her enormous grief; not only did it make her stand out like a sore thumb in the high school where she was now enrolled, but it made her look so much older that as an adult, when she came across old photographs of herself, she winced. But at the time she felt that this was a thing she must do.

When Helen began coming home immediately after school each day, her mother questioned her. "Don't you have cheerleading practice?" she asked, knowing what a large part of Helen's life this had formerly been.

"No," Helen answered quietly. "I would have to participate in activities on Friday night."

Mrs. Sanford ached to send Helen to an Adventist boarding academy, but they were barely able to hold the family together. There was simply no money. As Helen declined nominations for class offices and fund-raising activities and was at home by herself night after night, weekend after weekend, her mother's heart was bruised at the sight of the lonely, blue-eyed, earnest young girl.

"Must following Christ be so hard?" she whispered to herself.

The house, so long bursting with exuberant young manhood, was now largely silent. Harry had married. The young uncles had moved out, and even though they had been treated as members of the family, they seldom visited anymore because of the changed life style. From a full, happy, busy house, Helen went to a quiet, lonely home with only her parents, for now Marvin was having such difficulty in standing for the faith he too had espoused that his parents had decided that he must attend the boarding academy in Lodi, California. Ben Sanford decreed that Helen must go also. It was only fair, he said.

"She cannot be so lonely and isolated as she is now," he told his wife. "Let's rent out part of the house, and with that money and what the two of them can earn, perhaps they can stay in school in Lodi for a while."

Helen was horrified. "We can't give up our own home!" she cried, her voice trembling, tears gathering in her blue eyes. "I love our home."

But her mother and father had suffered silent anguish at the narrowing of Helen's life. They were concerned lest her loneliness cause her to turn her back on God. Her special, deep consecration was too precious to be risked.

An advertisement was put in the paper, offering most of the house, completely furnished, for rent. Lodi Academy was contacted. Helen and Marvin's meager possessions were packed. The train reservations were made. In spite of herself, Helen's heart beat high with anticipation. In just another day she would be part of a happy, loving, young Christian group. She would be able to participate in all their activities. She would not need to hold back at all. She could throw herself into every activity, and even though she would need to work as many hours as possible, there would still be the association in the dormitory with the other girls, along with morning and evening worships and chapels and—oh, it would all be so wonderful!

The morning dawned. Helen jumped from her bed, her fingers flying as she dressed. She ran into the living room—and stopped dead still. There sat her father, his head in his hands. His whole demeanor suggested such despair that Helen's heart began to beat wildly.

"What's the matter, Daddy?" she exclaimed, rushing to his side.

He could hardly speak. "Mother has gotten terribly, terribly sick," he told her. "I don't think you can go off and leave her. I don't know what's the matter with her."

This can't be happening! was the refrain running through

Helen's mind. It can't be true! But when she went into her mother's room, looked at the pale, suffering face on the pillow, and felt her mother's thin hand grasp her strong, young hand, she knew with a sick certainty that she could not leave her. With one imperceptible quiver of her chin, she said goodbye to her hopes and dreams.

"Mother, I wouldn't dream of going to Lodi," she soothed, kneeling down beside the bed. "I'm going to stay right here and take care of you."

Etta Sanford was caught between her terrible need and her sorrow for Helen.

"Perhaps I'll be better tomorrow," she whispered weakly. "Then you can go and you won't really miss much school." But she and Helen both knew that Helen would never go to Lodi Academy. However, Helen was determined that Marvin should go as planned. She stood at the door and waved goodbye to him as he and her father climbed into the car. Out of her mother's sight, she let the hot tears slide down her cheeks, now and again wiping them away with her hand. She must not let her mother know she had been crying. She crept into the bathroom and held a cold, wet washcloth to her eyes. Only when she felt that she had her voice under perfect control did she enter her mother's room and cheerfully announce, "Now I'm going to clean you up and fix you some breakfast."

Then there was the unpacking of all the things she'd packed so happily. She had to make arrangements to reenter her high school—and help her father get the house ready for the people who'd rented it. Marvin's bills would have to be taken care of, and besides, they had promised the house to a family of four, with the understanding that they would retain one room at the back of the house and a pantry; they would share the bathroom with the renters. All their personal possessions had to be taken from the front of the house and stored in boxes in the cellar. Their cooking would be done on a little coal-oil stove in a little pantry.

When the arrangements were completed, Helen gazed around the tiny room with a heart of lead. How could the three of them exist in these conditions? Life had been hard before; now it would be almost unendurable.

"Mother," she said, "I feel that I have to have one little private corner. If it's all right with you, I'm going to buy some muslin at the dime store and curtain off the back porch so it can be my private place. I saw some material for seven cents a yard."

Her mother answered, "Oh, Helen—I wish things could be different for you."

Surprised by this unexpected tenderness, Helen swallowed the lump in her throat.

For several years, Helen's "room" was the curtained-off porch. Though she had always been warm, friendly, and outgoing, attracting friends like a magnet, she withdrew into herself, too proud to accept invitations to the homes of her friends when she could not reciprocate. She could not invite a girlfriend for a meal served on a card table and cooked on a two-burner stove. She was never sure of the condition of the communal bathroom.

"Sometimes I don't even like our renters!" she burst out one evening as the three of them huddled around the card table, eating their simple meal. "They're living in our house where we should be living!"

"But they're paying for the house," her father reminded her. "Marvin is doing well at Lodi Academy, and that's what we were hoping for."

Actually, the renters were orderly, mannerly people—but they were Pentecostal, and from time to time, at night, the "gift of tongues" would come upon them, causing them to erupt into a great cacophony of sound. Helen dreaded these incidents.

Her strange religion (from her classmates' viewpoint), her inability to invite her friends to her home, her old-fashioned, unbecoming hairdo, and her refusal to join in the Friday and

Saturday school activities of sports, orchestra, chorus, and debating society left only one avenue open to her. She decided that she would study feverishly, ceaselessly.

"Maybe someday I can be secretary to a minister. Why, perhaps I might even be able to *marry* a minister!" she told her father, in a sudden upsurge of spirits. She attacked her shorthand and typing with fierce determination, refusing ever to turn in a typing assignment that wasn't perfect, though at times tears of frustration filled her eyes. Her high school counselor had convinced her that secretarial skills would be her best avenue toward employment in the depression-ridden world.

Sabbaths were spent at church. On Sundays she got up early, ate a few bites, then walked across the city of Reno to a rancher's home, the latter ranching during the week and coming to his house infrequently. When he came, however, he made no attempt to clean off his muddy boots or clothes before coming into the house. It was always incredibly dirty. Helen's arrangement was that she worked as hard as she could for four hours, never pausing for a long breath; then she walked the entire route home again. She was paid fifty cents an hour. Even had public transportation been available, she could not have afforded it. All her clothes and offerings, as well as money for her *Signs* list of subscribers, had to be provided from this two-dollar-a-week income.

The Sanford family, in attempting to observe Adventist dietary teachings, really had no idea of substitutions that must be made for the foods they had now discarded. Helen had been in the habit of eating large quantities of meat. As she entered her teens she usually drank four cups of coffee per day. Now all this stimulating food was gone. Her body craved something (she didn't know quite what), and so she and her parents began eating large quantities of sweets, relying on the quick energy sugar produces. But for Helen this depleted diet, coupled with her crushing loneliness, produced such a deep depression that it became difficult for her to push herself through the long daily tasks.

The depths of her despair became clear when she almost drowned at a church picnic. Unable to swim, she'd been persuaded into the deep waters of Donner Lake by an older woman who'd insisted that she could tow her across the lake. When her head kept going under, Helen panicked. Then it was downhill all the way, with the struggling, the frantic gasps for air, the rising to the surface momentarily, then sinking again. Suddenly the water around her began to feel like warm, caressing feathers. Lights flashed in front of her eyes. Helen had a warm, secure feeling. She knew she was drowning, but she did not feel afraid or even regretful. Oh, it isn't so bad to die like this, she thought drowsily and dreamily, for the next thing I will see will be Jesus coming. I won't have to be lonely anymore and have no young friends and I won't have to turn down boys who like me and I won't ever be poor again and not have the things that other kids have.

When Helen regained consciousness on the shore, in the arms of a young man in the church who was home on vacation, for a few moments she wasn't sure whether she was glad or sorry. It had all seemed so simple there in the engulfing, overwhelming water.

Like any other young girl, Helen had become conscious of the opposite sex in the questioning, poised-for-flight manner of that time. She certainly enjoyed smiling across a classroom at attractive boys with all the power of her hyacinth-blue eyes, and she experienced a delightful shiver down her spine when they smiled back. But she never let the smiles develop into anything else.

"How could I accept dates?" she said to her father. "I don't dance or go to the movies or to sports things on Friday night or Sabbath. And I can't bring a boy here to this one room."

But God remained the central figure in Helen's life, and her religion the center around which everything else revolved. She was very active in the church. She was, in fact, "the young people" of the church. The few others were in boarding school. Lonely people often drift together; in Helen's case, this meant that the few unattached older or sick clutched at her youth and vitality feverishly. There was one woman whose husband had left her, and who poured into the innocent ears of the 16-year-old intimate details of her marriage that Helen should never have heard and was horrified at hearing.

Helen had been paying for one subscription to *Signs of the Times* out of her meager funds, following the suggestion of the pastor. She also paid twenty-five cents a week to the Sabbath school as her offering. But the *Signs* subscription somehow seemed a more tangible endeavor, for she took the copy each week and left it at the house on the corner. Later, after she had been away from Reno for some time, the man on the corner was baptized. He said, "I was very interested in the Bible and in religion. Every time I would be studying a certain subject and praying for light, Helen seemed to leave a copy of the *Signs,* and there would be just what I needed in it to enlighten me." Always Helen was the backbone of the church music "staff," improving her skills constantly with the full repertoire of Adventist hymns.

But a few months of brightness presented themselves when a beautiful young girl from Pacific Union College came to Reno as a secretary in the conference office. Mary had been engaged to a fine young dentist who had no interest in Seventh-day Adventism. Acting on the advice of others, she had broken her engagement—and also her heart. She was so desolate, so lonely, that Helen felt her own situation was almost good by comparison. She spent her free time with Mary during that period. One of their quiet activities during one summer was to walk downtown to the public library. As they strolled along on one of these walks, they talked about the difficulty of Christian living. They discussed their great desire to honor Christ in all their actions. Then Mary made, for Helen, a surprising statement.

"The hardest thing for me was giving up novel reading."

Helen stopped still in the middle of the sidewalk. Why, her family had literally been nurtured on novels, with her mother's voracious appetite for reading! Many of the novels had been read aloud, with the entire family commenting on the plot and characters. Could this possibly be wrong?

"I'm not sure I agree with that," Helen told her new friend, with the frankness and sincerity that was her usual approach to a problem.

"Study *Messages to Young People* and see how you feel," was Mary's gentle suggestion.

Helen started her study that very night. With a prayer for guidance and an open mind, shortly she decided that she must confine herself in the future to biography, true adventure, and other true stories.

"How will I manage in my English class?" she asked herself. After thinking for a moment, she realized that she must go to her English teacher and explain her position and offer to do extra reading, if necessary, but to be allowed to substitute true books for novels.

Startled at first by her request, her current teacher gazed at her thoughtfully. "Helen, you're one of my best students. You do all your work as fully and conscientiously as possible. I am sure you have a good reason for your decision. And I'm going to grant your request."

Grateful, Helen worked twice as hard to live up to her teacher's expectations. She made the same arrangements with subsequent English teachers—and finally became something of an authority on the life, work, and times of John Muir.

By this time Helen's artistic skills were well-known to the conference. For camp meetings she usually made all the booklets, decorations, and other aids used in the children's tent. She hadn't planned to attend camp meeting during one particular summer, since a dream had come true in that an opportunity to join an art class taught by a university art teacher had opened up. During that first session of the class, held in the foothills near Reno, Helen's eyes were opened to so much beauty that she was transfixed. All her life she'd longed to draw, to paint. Her hands ached for the feel of the brush—hands that in her short life had held scrubbing boards, irons, cooking utensils, and gardening tools. Now at last she would discover whether or not she might have a future in the art world. Was her talent big enough?

On the way home she was in a dream world—a world that shattered abruptly when her mother exclaimed, as she entered the door, "Helen, the people at the Lake Tahoe camp meeting have been frantically trying to get in touch with you. They are desperate for an organist for the children's tent."

"But I just started my art class. I can't possibly go!" Helen cried.

"Then tell them that," her mother urged. "But you must call them back in order to be polite."

With every intention of refusing the offer, Helen placed the call. But the persuasion on the other end of the line was too strong. "After all," she said to herself, "Jesus is coming soon. He needs me at camp meeting more than He needs me in an art class. There will be other chances to study art."

But there never were until it was almost too late.

Helen loved, as always, the spiritual feast of the meetings, the feeling that God was near in an unusual way. The camp meeting, however, brought heartache, for her cousin Dorothea announced that after many struggles she had decided to be baptized. When Dorothea's mother was informed, she rushed to Lake Tahoe from Reno, a distance of about forty miles, threw Dorothea's things together, and took her home. Because of Helen's different life style the sisterlike relationship was never the same, and this was another bereavement for Helen.

Later Helen was one of the mainstays of the first junior

camp ever held in the area, acting as counselor, assistant cook, nursemaid, and playground supervisor. "Helen, you always seem to be where the hard work is," her father teased her.

Then it was graduation time. School was over. Helen had to find a job. In 1932, with the great depression gripping the land, there was no thought of college.

CHAPTER 5

Lonely Days

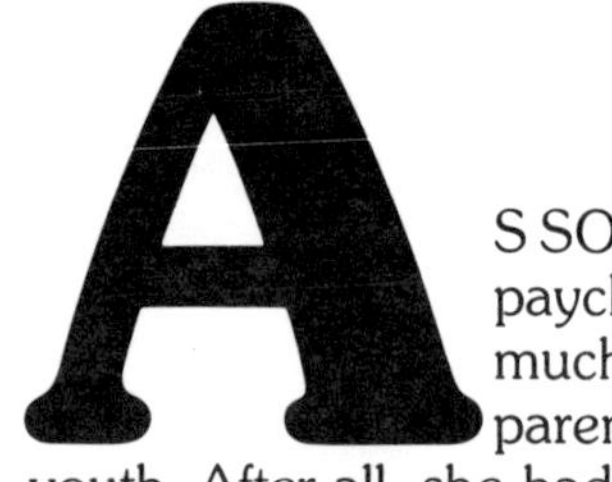

S SOON as I get a job and have a regular paycheck coming in, things will be so much better for us," Helen told her parents with the same high hopes of youth. After all, she had been assured by her teachers that secretarial training was the key that would unlock her future. Now the first day of the rest of her life had dawned.

It was a sadder, wearier, and wiser girl who returned home after that first day of walking street after street, of entering office after office, only to be told, "Sorry. We can't take on any new people. If the depression lessens . . ."

When the days slipped by and a week had passed, and then another, and Helen was still jobless, she came to her father with tears in her eyes. "Now I know how you've felt all this time, Daddy," she said as she hugged him. "I don't know how you've kept us going and how you've endured constantly working as a salesman when times are so hard and with no regular paycheck."

He hugged his "little" girl. "It hasn't been easy, but the Lord is good, and the best day of my life was my baptism," he asserted stoutly. "After all, the things in this world aren't the final ones."

Helen never, in her wildest conjectures, had visualized that the whole summer would pass and still she would be unemployed; but it did. She could not continue to exist with no pattern or purpose. Was her life over before it had really begun?

"I know what I'll do—I'll enroll at high school for some advanced work in shorthand," she decided aloud, as she and her parents discussed her dilemma. "Then I'll have something to do." This plan worked well for several months. In fact, when the high school administrative offices needed extra help from time to time, they hired Helen. This bit of money helped augment her weekly two-dollar cleaning money.

But sickness, the horror of Helen's life, again intruded. Harry's wife also contracted tuberculosis. There were now two small girls in their home, at some distance from Reno. In desperation, Harry phoned. "What in the world am I going to do?" he asked. "Can't Helen come and hold the fort?"

There seemed no question that this was Helen's duty as a Christian and as Harry's sister. But she had known so much sickness. She had never really known anything else. She did her best, heavy-hearted, with the endless routine learned in childhood and youth.

Then life came up with a surprise. A long-distance call came in for Helen. Long-distance calls weren't usual in those days, except in emergencies. As Harry listened to Helen's responses, his curiosity grew.

"No, I can't," she said. "Yes, I do have the training. I think I could do the work. But I can't leave here."

As soon as she had hung up, he pounced on her. "What was that all about?" he demanded.

When Helen told him that the conference office, now in Salt Lake City, needed a secretary, because of the resignation of their present secretary, he announced firmly, "Of course you'll take the job. This is what you have been waiting for."

"But, Harry," Helen protested, "it will be only temporary. When the school year is out, they plan to call a girl from La Sierra Junior College or from Pacific Union College. They don't think just a high school graduate will fill the bill permanently."

He brushed her objections aside. He must have realized that his little sister hadn't had much of a chance in life.

"Just get your foot in the door and see what happens.

Now get on the phone and call them back immediately," he told her. She did.

One thing Helen wouldn't be taking along to Salt Lake City was her long hair with the rebellious knot on her neck. After years of struggling with it, one day, as she walked by a barbershop, she had, on impulse, gone in and determinedly directed the barber to cut her hair. He had obliged, all too thoroughly, with no attempt at styling. When her father had seen her, his face had turned bright red. At last he had blurted out, "Well, if you aren't one horrible-looking mess!" Now she had finally learned to curl and tame her hair, but not without many struggles. Then "frizzy" permanents became the order of the day.

The seven-hundred-mile train trip was thrilling to a young girl who had so little opportunity for travel. Her heart was beating high with anticipation. A whole new world was suddenly opening up before her! What would it be like? Would she be able to do the work? Could she manage on whatever salary they would pay her? Could it be that the church in Salt Lake City might number some eligible Adventist boys among their members?

Alas for the dreams of youth! With the sublime disregard for personal preference in matters affecting the young that was the hallmark of that era, Helen was met at the train by one of the conference officials, told that she would receive fourteen dollars per week and that arrangements had already been made for her housing.

"You will room and board with a lady and her daughter," the official told the shy, tall, blue-eyed girl, who was too overwhelmed even to ask questions.

After the drive to the conference office to show Helen its location, he deposited her, with her battered suitcases, on the steps of a run-down house and left. On weak knees she went up the steps, rang the bell, and finally was admitted into one of the strangest households she had ever known or would ever know.

The house was overrun by a cat, an animal Helen had never encountered because of her father's violent allergy to cat fur. Helen was prepared to make friends with the feline, but not to eat off the same dishes with the cat—the dishes unwashed. Not only was the cat fed in the sink where the dishes were washed, but after it had licked the dishes dry the latter were put into the cupboards for family use! The entire house reeked of cheap cat food—fish. Helen, used to immaculate cleanliness, was sickened. She realized that she must move as soon as possible. But first she must get her bearings in a conference office where she was the only secretary, the only stenographer, the only "gofer." It became clear almost immediately that her status as "only" a high school graduate would be the excuse for denigrating and criticizing mistakes made in ignorance!

At first, though, she had such high hopes that nothing seemed difficult. On her own, she found other living quarters—three unconnected rooms in an upstairs house with the bottom floor occupied by a young colporteur and his wife and baby. Helen had no bathroom, only a toilet in a closet. She probably could have asked the colporteur wife if she could take an occasional bath in her tub, but she was shy and proud, and besides, the home philosophy rang through her mind: "Helen, don't you ever, ever ask anybody for anything. What you can't get for yourself, do without."

She had sacks of coal delivered upstairs for her little "trash burner" stove, the only heating device, which left the rooms as cold in winter as they were hot in summer. She did her washing in the sink in one of the rooms and took "baths" in that same sink.

For this "mansion" Helen paid ten dollars a month, out of her fourteen-dollar-a-week salary. Her inexperience made her feel fourteen dollars was a very generous amount. Pathetically grateful to have a job, she never thought it strange that she carried, with no complaint, all the work of a more experienced secretary.

The Salt Lake City church didn't have many young people. As in Reno, the youth of the church went away to boarding school; they canvassed during the summers. Now, with a steady income, Helen began to feel, almost from the first week, a thirst for more education that was with her every minute of the day. But no one ever said to her, "Helen, you should go on to college." It seemed to be taken for granted that she would always remain just what she then was. To herself she resolved that no matter what it took, no matter what sacrifices were necessary, she would one day go to an Adventist college. In the meantime, she would throw herself totally into her work; she would be the very best secretary they had ever had. She would also join in the activities of the small church with all her might. She'd forget about her high hopes of not being so lonely anymore. After all, now she had college to look forward to—sometime. She could manage without spending much more than her rent and for the most minimal food. Most people ate too much, didn't they? Well, she would put herself on a restricted diet, which would be good for her figure—well, maybe not too good, since she was already so thin, but certainly good for her health. Things would work out.

Helen had no trouble with spelling, typing, and shorthand. English had been one of her best subjects. But she had a little difficulty understanding all the varied, unrelated duties that were assigned to her. For instance, she was expected to walk a mile to pick up the mail in the morning when all the men were out of town, no matter what the weather. It could have been delivered to the office, by special arrangement, but she was told, "The extra walk will be good for you. Just be sure you're here at the office on time!"

When the conference office moved to a new building, she was told it was her job to clean out the toilets the workmen had used. She also had to clean the paint off the windows and wash them until they sparkled. There was an upstairs room in the office where colporteurs stayed when they came to the conference office. "It is your responsibility to keep the bed freshly made up and the room clean," one of her bosses told her. When the janitor suddenly walked off the job, Helen was appointed to take his place—temporarily, of course. It was surprising how long "temporary" turned out to be. She shoveled snow from walks in the winter if the men were gone. After all, it was "good for her"!

When Helen had been working in the conference office only a couple of weeks and was still terrified that she might not succeed, she was told to type a book order that would run more than a hundred pounds. "Order them to be shipped to us by freight," the official commanded.

Helen was puzzled. She really had no information regarding ways books could be sent. She didn't know that such a thing as "freight" existed. It seemed logical—the only solution, actually—to type "parcel post" on the order. She was afraid to ask any more questions. In due time the books arrived, carrying a shipping charge of four dollars.

"Four dollars!" exploded the conference official. "That's much more than it would have been by freight. Now I am going to teach you a lesson, Helen. I am going to take the four dollars out of this week's paycheck."

Helen felt the tears rising to her eyes and the lump coming into her throat. With only fourteen dollars to begin with, and her ambition to save, this seemed hard. But she choked back the rebellious words that sprang to her lips. Underneath, though, she could not help feeling that the official could have looked over the slip when she finished typing it, and, in view of her inexperience, headed off the problem.

Since the conference officials were in and out of the office between their travels throughout the conference, they expected Helen to be ready to take dictation at any hour from 8:00 A.M. on. It was not at all unusual for one or more of the men to dictate until ten or eleven at night, then jump into their cars and head for home, leaving the teen-aged girl to get home in the dark the best way she could.

"I'm sorry I can't offer you a ride, but it just wouldn't look right," one of the officials told her as he pulled out of the lot.

Numberless times Helen crept down the middle of the street, walking the mile to her apartment, singing under her breath, " 'I'll go where You want me to go, dear Lord,' " and jumping, her heart in her throat, at every shadow that moved. The night walks were especially frightening in the middle of snowstorms.

The literature evangelist leader, a most enterprising man, conceived the idea of sending the colporteurs' sales to each customer C.O.D. to save time. Just whose time was saved, Helen was never sure, for this meant that she must stay nearly every night until ten, at least, wrapping the books and making out C.O.D. orders. As if that were not enough, by the time the C.O.D. books arrived, a Mormon bishop would have heard that a "heretic" was loose among his flock and would have brought considerable pressure to bear on the hapless book purchaser. This meant that great sacks of books would come back, rejected. Then Helen had to unwrap those, record them in the journal, and get them back on the proper shelves. Credit memos had to be written out for each one. Helen, who did not consider math her strong point, found the entire proceeding a nightmare—almost literally.

It was then the custom for all the church school children to take final examinations that were corrected in the conference office, graded, then recorded, with the records being kept in the office. In addition to her other duties, this also fell to Helen's lot. During one summer she was so snowed under that if one of the Pacific Union College colporteur boys had not volunteered to help her, she might have finally gone under. She worried for fear he had not graded the tests properly. "But after all," she told herself, "he's a college student and knows more than I do." She just wanted to be sure that no child was failed who should have passed. It wasn't an age of "automatic promotion." The children who failed the tests simply did not go on to the next grade.

Helen had become a vital part of the little Salt Lake City church, making the goal devices and other interest devices for the children, playing the piano or organ for most of the meetings, and helping out in an effort the conference president held. She developed a lifelong interest in the sanctuary because of Elder W. D. Frazee's tent effort. As she gazed at the beautiful model of the sanctuary that Elder Frazee used, she felt transported. How logical and beautiful it all was! How it all fitted together! How fortunate she was to have heard the beautiful message of God's truth and to be preparing for Christ's soon coming. Nothing seemed to matter when compared to that central fact.

During that first cold, snowy, overworked winter, Helen developed such severe tonsillitis that she was sick all the time. But she took not one day off from work. She would arrive in the morning after her cold walk achy, feverish, with a throat so sore that it seemed filled with ground glass. Finally she felt so miserable that she confided her distress to a doctor from Loma Linda who was attempting to establish a self-supporting clinic in the area. One glance at her tonsils and he was horrified.

"You must have these things removed immediately," he told her. "They are almost dripping with pus."

"But I have no money," Helen told him.

"Just come down to my office and I will take them out for you for five dollars," he assured the young girl, thinking that the minimal charge would save her pride. He realized that he was dealing with a person who expected no favors from life.

They made their arrangements. On the next Friday afternoon Helen was driven to his office by the teacher and his wife. She sat down in a chair and was draped with a sheet. The doctor injected her neck and throat with Novocain liberally, then waited a few minutes. As Helen saw him approaching with what seemed to her a steel rod ending in a wire loop, she was so terrified that her eyes opened as wide as saucers—then she determinedly squeezed them shut. This was no time to back out, she scolded herself. In short order the deed was done. The offending bits of tissue resided on the doctor's tray, not in Helen's throat. In later years she shuddered as she thought of what could have happened—hemorrhage, infection, and so on. But ignorance is often bliss. The schoolteacher and his wife had a little 13-year-old girl living with them so she could attend the church school. Concerned about Helen, they sent the child home with her to Helen's upstairs apartment—"just in case." And in the early evening, the downstairs tenants sent up a bowl of hot mushroom soup. Anyone who tries to eat hot, highly seasoned soup a few hours after a tonsillectomy will sympathize with Helen's suffering. But she went to church as usual on Sabbath and even nibbled a few bites of apples and popcorn at the schoolteacher's house on Saturday night. When it was all over and her throat had healed, she wrote and told her parents about the surgery. It wouldn't have occurred to her to worry her frail mother. From the beginning Helen's father had trained the three children to keep their troubles to themselves and to cope with life.

The small church in Salt Lake City was having a very hard time financially. A board meeting was held. "We'll have Helen Sanford move into the front part of the schoolteacher's house," they decided. "Then we'll have the income from her rent." And so Helen moved again, to a run-down little house on the lot behind the church, owned by the congregation. There were three rooms more or less at the back of the house and two at the front, which would be Helen's "apartment." She would share the bath with the schoolteacher and his wife. The furniture was old and dreadful; there was a little gas stove, but it threw out so much moisture that condensation formed on the walls and windows, and the air took on a menacing smell. There was also a coal stove. Helen had to get up very early in winter to get a coal fire started, bank it, then walk to work through the snow and wind—and return late at night in the dark, only to find her rooms icy cold. The fire could never be banked to last all day.

Since there was no place for Helen to store her kindling and coal, her father and mother scraped together money to make a special trip from Reno to see whether they couldn't improve her living conditions just a bit. He hauled box after wooden box from the grocery stores, chopped them up into kindling, and stacked them in a storage room of the church basement, having gotten the consent of the officials for this. He hauled in what he thought was a large supply of coal. He and her mother went back to Reno, happy in the thought that Helen would have fuel for most of the winter.

Then a meeting of several days' duration was held in the church. At the conclusion of the meeting, when Helen went to check on her fuel supply, it was totally gone. It had been used by those conducting the meeting; she faced the winter with no kindling, no coal. For once her brave composure deserted her and she wrote her father, feeling that she could not exist without his loving sympathy.

Though he said little, except to reassure her that she would manage and that the Lord would help her, in later years he told Helen what a severe test of faith it had been for him.

"To think that those men would be so unconcerned about a young girl angered me terribly," he said. "And beyond that, they were taking property that was not theirs. If I could have done so, I would have brought you home immediately. But you know how it was—you felt you were so needed in that Mormon stronghold and struggling small conference."

Helen assured him that she had managed somehow, someway.

Another heartache coming about the same time had to do with Marvin's wedding. This important family event was to take place during the Christmas holidays. Helen fearfully approached the official from whom she would need permission to return home. "My brother wants me there so badly," she told him. "He'll never get over it if I'm not. May I go?"

He didn't hesitate a moment. "Certainly *not!*" he roared. "The auditor will be coming right after Christmas. The last thing in the world we're going to do is have you out of the office. Just forget it."

Hurt, bewildered, uncomprehending, she stumbled out of his office and back to her desk. She wrote the sad letter telling her family that she would not be home. Each time she heard a Christmas carol, her heart ached more sharply. Surely—surely something would happen. But it didn't.

On Christmas Day Helen sat alone at the piano in the cold church, playing hymns, as the slow tears coursed down her cheeks.

None of the conference officials and their wives invited her to Christmas dinner. Only the kind schoolteacher and his wife remembered that an 18-year-old girl needs a happy holiday; they did their best.

Helen soon learned that the conference officials, to say nothing of the church members, had strong opinions as to what a single secretary could and couldn't do. She couldn't play tennis with the publishing secretary and his wife, when the latter sat on the sidelines and watched. It "didn't look good." She really couldn't associate with young men at all. Helen wondered just how the sexes ever got together!

She had a very decided reason for wondering. A new, exciting set of circumstances had developed. A group of young male students had come to Utah from Pacific Union College to canvass for the summer. During the depression, the conferences had hit upon the scheme of offering scholarships of varying amounts to students who spent an entire summer canvassing. This was a mutually beneficial arrangement since it provided for the distribution of Adventist literature while helping the students with scanty resources to obtain a Christian education.

Like homing pigeons, the boys discovered Helen—tall, graceful, willowy, blue-eyed Helen, so full of life and vitality, so burdened with responsibility, so appealing. Used to a houseful of boys in her growing-up years, she bandied words with them, took their teasing gracefully, listened to their problems, and often wrapped books for them until late at night.

Helen met Stanley Jefferson during that summer.

He and Wayne Andrews and several other boys complained loudly in her presence that they were starving. They had to eat when and where they could. They didn't have enough money for a decent restaurant meal. Oh, for a home-cooked dinner.

Spontaneously and automatically Helen responded, her blue eyes twinkling. "If you'll buy the food, you can bring it to my place and cook yourselves a dinner."

Elated, they made the arrangements. Alas, even though a single woman was taking care of the schoolteacher's apartment for the summer and was with the group the whole time, the very next morning the conference treasurer called Helen into his office. He was so stern, so condemnatory, so threatening, that Helen broke down and sobbed brokenheartedly. For this one brief hour she had been a "normal" girl, lighthearted and free. The evening had been entirely innocent. Was she never to have any fun in her life? From then on she never invited any of the colporteur boys even to stop at her door. But during the second summer, when Stanley returned to Utah, she took her courage in her hands, and when he asked her to go for a ride in James Lee's car—a Model A Ford with a rumble seat—she said Yes. (James and his date accepted the "rumble.") The big treat of the evening were the candy bars the boys stopped and bought.

Stanley started creating moments when their paths would cross. He tried to convey to her—at least she timidly thought he did—that he wanted to know her better. And when he went back to college that year, he began writing to her.

In 1936 the Nevada-Utah Conference bought a large, old three-story stone house with a two-story barn on the property and opened an academy there in Salt Lake City. The top floor was to house the girls; the main floor, with one large room and one smaller room, was the classroom area. The downstairs was used for the kitchen, dining room, and the two rooms that housed the principal and his wife. The boys were assigned the barn, which was only a stone's throw from the main building and from the girls' rooms. There was a great deal of communication between the two areas.

After many committee meetings and much mysterious whispering and planning, Helen was called into the office of the conference president. "Miss Sanford," he said, "we are going to give you the privilege of being preceptress of the new academy. You will live there with the girls and be responsible for their conduct at all times. We will hold you accountable for whatever happens."

Helen was stunned. She was speechless for a moment. Then she burst out, "But I don't want to be a preceptress! I'm a secretary! Do you mean you're firing me from my job here?"

"Certainly not" was his cool rejoinder. "You'll put in your regular eight hours here each day, then walk to the academy—it's only a mile—and take over there. You can share a room with one of the girls and save space."

For once Helen felt that she really couldn't cope. And when he went on to say that she'd have to pay for the privilege of working and living there, Helen fled to a phone. She made an unprecedented long-distance call to her parents, who were understandably outraged.

"You're doing the work of three people now," her father said. "Mother and I will drive over there and try to block this plan."

They were no match for the eloquent officials, however, who declared that the whole academy venture was a "test of faith" and a "mission field," and that it would need the full endeavor of every person for it to succeed. Beaten, Ben Sanford held out for one last item. "Helen must have a sunny room to herself," he declared adamantly, and the administrator agreed. The "sunny room" turned out to be a dark northeast room in which the sun never penetrated, and as time went on, one of the dormitory girls was found to be so unpleasant that no one else would room with her. So Helen "inherited" her, body odor and all. But Helen learned to love and appreciate her for her good qualities.

Now her life fell into a new pattern. She had to be up very early for her private devotions. Then, in quick succession, she was to ring the bell, herd the girls downstairs to breakfast, eat with them, then fly out the door to walk the mile to the office and arrive on time. Sometimes she would have to run the last half-mile. This was a particularly snowy winter in Salt Lake City. One morning she found that only a milk truck had broken through the crust of the snow before her. When she arrived at the office, snow was so packed in the top of her galoshes that one little spot on her leg had turned white; it was frostbitten. No one else arrived for hours; some did not arrive at all.

At five o'clock, breathless, her heart beating fast from her rush to get all the most pressing work done, she reversed her step for the mile run back to the academy. After supper it was her responsibility to supervise the study hall in the classrooms and keep the girls *and* the boys quiet. At bedtime she rang another bell, which was the signal for the students to turn off their lights and get to bed promptly. Unfortunately, their interpretation of *promptly* differed widely from hers. When finally they were quiet, she could then write letters to her parents—or Stanley—and make necessary repairs on her few clothes. On Sundays she had to wash—by hand. And on Sabbaths she had to continue to supervise the students, being extra-careful to see that nothing untoward happened when they were less regimented than on weekdays.

During the past two years Helen had continued to put in the bank every cent that she did not need—and many that she did need. In her new role, she agonized over the fact that she was being charged $22.50 for room and board, which meant that her living cost her more than it previously had—yet she was working two full-time jobs. When she asked whether she might use one of the school's pianos to practice on, she was told that she was welcome to do so—for a fee of $2.50 a month.

Helen took a deep interest in the students, some of them not much younger than she. Many had not been used to established rules of conduct in their homes. It seemed like a hopeless task to instill in them a love for God and His principles. Sometimes, late at night, when they were all bedded down, Helen would walk out in the snow, salty tears mingling with the snowflakes, weeping for the headstrong students, for the drabness of her existence and for—she knew not what. There was a vast, deep longing in her heart. She wanted to be loved and cherished. Would she ever know this most beautiful of human experiences?

The letters from Stanley continued to arrive regularly. She began to wait for them eagerly, uneasy when it seemed that a longer interval than usual had elapsed. In the quiet of the night, she would remember how he looked—tall, well-built, brown-haired, brown-eyed. She would remember what he was like—courteous, gentle, gallant. Was it too much to hope?

Apparently it was. During the last summer she was in Salt Lake City, Helen heard that Stanley had abruptly repudiated his strong Christian commitment, was discouraged spiritually, and was associated with a pretty worldly crowd.

The correspondence ceased. Another bereavement, another abandonment.

CHAPTER 6

Engaged!

THROUGH that last long winter in Salt Lake City, a conviction grew in Helen's mind that eventually emerged as a fierce determination: It was now or never. She must go to college. If she did not, she would become so enmeshed in her office job, the school job, and her church work that she would never extricate herself. She visualized herself twenty-five years in the future, still toiling away until late at night, by now a fixture in the conference office, though, hopefully, not in the dormitory. Surely life had many new horizons for her to explore. There was so much she wanted to learn. Her need for young people her own age at times seemed almost like a hunger for physical food. Month by slow month her savings grew. "Going to college" became the central focus of her future plans.

When she opened her bank book one day and looked at the total of her savings—$350—she made her decision. "I am going to Pacific Union College for the next school year," she whispered to herself. "If they will give me lots of work, with what I have saved, I know that I can get through at least one year."

Then she knelt and prayed, joy flooding her heart. She was full of gratitude to God for having watched over her in her lonely state, in having kept her purpose strong and clear, and for having preserved her health.

She could hardly wait to write to Pacific Union College. Then came the waiting for their reply. How could it take so long? Had her letter gotten lost in the mail? She scolded herself for her impatience. After all, she wasn't the only would-be student they had to deal with. It must be a complicated situation, with so many students needing work in the depression days. When the letter finally arrived, eager as she had been to receive it, she could hardly summon the courage to open it. What if they said there was no work for a young woman with finely honed secretarial skills? Actually, she'd told them she'd work anywhere, do anything. As long as she could be in college, her daily work mattered little.

The words leaped out from the page. *Yes!* They had work for her. *Yes!* She would be going to college.*

She must tell the conference officials in plenty of time, although, since they had finally added another girl to the office staff after she had been appointed preceptress at the academy, she knew that the work would go on without too much of a crisis. She was not letting anyone down.

Her employers weren't as happy about her future plans as she had expected. She had thought they'd congratulate her on wanting more education and commend her for having saved her money so rigorously. But their congratulations were tepid. Then she was called into one of the offices.

"Helen," one of the conference officials said solemnly, "I am sure you will want to leave a tangible gift here in this conference in appreciation for all the good things that have happened to you. This is a real mission field. You know how short of cash we are. We feel that you should make a twenty-five-dollar donation for the work here."

"Twenty-five dollars!" Helen gasped. "But I have such a little bit of money to see me through. I'll have to buy books and a few things for my room and I'll have to pay train fare to California and——"

He interrupted her sternly. "The Lord expects sacrifice from all of us," he told her.

Weakly Helen agreed. She didn't want to let the Lord

---

* She would be secretary to Dr. Mortensen, one of the science teachers, who was filling in as business manager that year. During her second year an experienced businessman and historian, Dr. Alvin W. Johnson, was business manager, and she was his secretary.

down. But when later she was matriculating at Pacific Union College, she realized that she could have taken another course if she had had that twenty-five dollars. Still, she didn't want to be selfish with her Lord. And she never regretted her gift, even when she learned that the official who had commanded her to give it owned a number of rental properties in the city.

Pacific Union College was, in those days, a unique institution, in that it provided its students with an almost totally controlled environment. Situated in the heart of an extinct volcano on top of Howell Mountain on the edge of Napa Valley, the college was in a strong position to resist secular trends with which its conservative faculty did not agree. First and foremost, the college was keenly aware of its role as a spiritual institution. Faculty members were dedicated to shaping every aspect of the young lives in their charge. There was strict supervision on the campus; easy association between the sexes was frowned upon; in fact, it was made very difficult by the rigid structure of rules and traditions. Just how young people were to meet their life partners was not a prime concern, though with the buoyancy of youth the students managed rather well. Faculty members took a personal interest in the students, made firm assessments of their probable futures, and did not hesitate to intrude themselves into the romantic relationships that developed.

A great emphasis was placed on the role of nature. A slogan of the college was "Where nature and revelation unite in education." The students were encouraged on Sabbath afternoons to hike to especially scenic spots in the mountains, always with chaperons. Study periods at night were strictly observed, with lights in Graf Hall, the girls' dormitory, being turned out by a central switch at nine-thirty. If the girls were not ready for lights out, they stumbled around in the dark with flashlights. The boys in Grainger Hall had a bit more freedom than their female counterparts, in that they were not required to sign out whenever they left the dormitory after six in the evening. All meals were taken in the dining room in Graf Hall. Six students were assigned to each table, with a young man appointed as the "host" and a young woman as the "hostess." Table assignments were changed about every six weeks; if a student was assigned to a table he disliked, with students he found uncongenial, there was nothing he could do but endure his misery. And one could never join another table unless he was the only student who appeared at his own. As romances flourished, this rule was broken from time to time, especially on weekends, to the great anguish of the matron, who regarded her rules on a par with those handed down from Sinai. "Couples" were never placed at the same table except when the news of a romance hadn't reached the matron's ears. But she seemed always up to the minute in that area.

One would naturally assume that the students would be miserably unhappy in such a restricted environment. Nothing could be further from the truth. Probably no other Adventist college inspired in its students a more fierce loyalty than did Pacific Union College. As a matter of fact, the students rather enjoyed the distinction of attending a college recognized far and wide as the most tightly disciplined of them all. To be a PUC-ite was considered a special category indeed. And always the students had the knowledge, the heartwarming realization, that the faculty *cared.* The outstanding dormitory deans, both now legends in their own times, Minnie E. Dauphinee (Roberts) and Walter B. Clark, inspired their charges to heights they would never otherwise have achieved.

Helen, used to intense self-discipline and the rigid structure of her life in Salt Lake City, found PUC paradise. None of the rules touched her, and so this was a little bit of heaven; this was what she had dreamed of and longed for. Even when she began to discover the slight imperfections beneath the surface, she was completely serene. God seemed nearer to her than she had ever dreamed possible.

Loving the outdoors with the strong intensity of her nature, Helen asked, soon after her arrival, whether she might work outdoors. The hilly slopes on which the college buildings were located were planted in vines. Flower beds were located at frequent intervals. "I'd love to spend my working time outdoors in all this beauty," she told them.

The college officials were shocked. Young women in the thirties did not work as gardeners, any more than they wore slacks. Young women worked in offices and schoolrooms and wore dresses. "Dr. Mortensen is expecting you," Helen was told. Used to obeying, she made no further objections.

Having known very little of the financial circumstances of the lives of other young people, it had never occurred to Helen that she might be assigned a roommate from a totally different economic sphere. As a matter of fact, Miss Dauphinee usually tried to avoid this kind of thing, since it was bound to cause a great deal of unhappiness. But it wasn't always possible to know just how affluent a background the students came from. As fate would have it, Helen's roommate was a girl from a wealthy family, a girl who had so many lovely clothes that the small closet literally bulged at the edges. Helen's pitifully few clothes were almost lost in her closet. The mainstay of her wardrobe was one suit of good-quality wool that her father had gotten for her at a time when he was selling suits. Helen had winced when she saw it, but her father had meant well. "This suit doesn't have one bit of style," she had told herself wryly. But the material was excellent, so she purchased several plain, tailored blouses to wear with the suit to attend classes. On Sabbath she wore the suit again, this time with a blouse she loved—a soft, feminine pink one. As for shoes, she had only two pairs to withstand the rigorous walking that was so much a part of being a PUC student, with the up-and-down campus requiring goatlike agility. It was hard on shoes. Her roommate went home often on weekends, always bringing back more clothes to crowd her closet further, though Helen knew her parents could well afford the money and the girl herself was kindhearted and generous. But the contrast was just too great. Miss Dauphinee changed roommates, but this time Helen was assigned another girl from a wealthy background, for specific reasons.

"You'll be a good influence on her, I know," Miss Dauphinee told Helen. "She's having a hard time adjusting to the rules. She's been used to so much more freedom."

Helen wasn't sure she wanted to be *thought* of as a "good influence"—though she certainly wanted to *be* one. When her new roommate found she really could not adjust to the rules and returned home, there was no other roommate available. Helen was alone—again. Actually, she could have roomed with the assistant dean, who already had one roommate; the price of the room would be somewhat less.

"It isn't that I don't like her—I just don't want to be thought of as one of the 'older' girls," Helen explained earnestly to Eileen Hare, one of her new friends. "Of course I know I am a few years older than the average freshman, but I certainly don't want to call attention to it!"

Eileen, exuberant, lively, irrepressible, agreed with her. "You deserve to have all the fun you can get!" she declared loyally.

Now Helen could hardly wait to get up each morning. Used as she was to early hours, the 5:45 A.M. rising bell held no terrors. It seemed to her that even her wiry hair benefited from the salubrious climate on Howell Mountain. It was a good thing, for no girl could appear in the worship room with curlers in her hair when the bell rang at six-fifteen. The first time Helen saw a crowd of girls fleeing toward the worship room to beat the tardy bell, snatching curlers from their hair as they ran, she burst out laughing. Later on, as she became busier and more tired, she even resorted to the same ploy once or twice herself.

Miss Dauphinee stopped her in the hall one day. Helen

could not know that her enormous, loving heart was touched by the tall, valiant, dedicated young girl, who so often had dark circles of fatigue under her eyes.

"Are you enjoying college as much as you thought you would, Helen?" she asked.

Helen's whole face burst into radiance. "Oh, it's so wonderful! I love everything about it. The classes are opening all sorts of new worlds to me, and the worships here in the dormitory are so inspiring, and the Friday-night meetings are so solemn and beautiful, and Sabbath is special, since I usually get to take a hike in the afternoon to some of the interesting nature places—" She stopped for breath.

"And you're making some lovely friends," Miss Dauphinee smiled. "Eileen Hare, Esther McVicker, Lorraine Moore—they are all splendid girls. You've chosen wisely." Then she paused for a moment. "Helen," she said, "I don't ever want to appear to interfere in my girls' lives. But a little bird told me that you and Mr. Jefferson were friends in Utah and that you corresponded for quite some time. But I haven't seen the two of you together, and I was wondering—"

She left the sentence in midair. Helen suppressed a smile at Miss Dauphinee's formality; never did she allude to the young men by their given names. Then Helen's blue eyes clouded over.

"Well," she began hesitantly, "you know that Stanley has kind of lost his way. When we were good friends, he was so earnest about his life's ambition to enter the ministry; he seemed to have such firm ideals. Here on the campus he's in a group that I wouldn't feel comfortable with—and actually, it was never a romance, but only a friendship," she finished sturdily.

Miss Dauphinee wasn't quite convinced. "Sometimes young people need friends to stand by them at critical times," she remarked quietly, then dropped the subject.

From the moment she had arrived at PUC, Helen had hoped against hope that Stanley had gotten past his rebellious frame of mind and that the two of them would somehow get together, in spite of the fact that they hadn't been corresponding for some time. "After all," she had told herself, "I can't believe he's forgotten me."

But since it had, in truth, never been a romance—not even one episode of holding hands—she armored herself in her girlish pride. Each time she would encounter Stan in the halls or on the campus, she had that heart-stopping sensation that he was as aware of her as she was of him. There was definitely electricity between the two of them—wasn't there? But even as she hugged to herself the warm thought that this was so, she sadly pushed aside any plans to further the attraction. When and if she married, it must not be to someone who was not as committed to God as she was. She couldn't even visualize a home where worship wouldn't be conducted, where the hope of a soon-coming Christ wasn't paramount, where Bible study wasn't a joy. And even as she told herself not to be ridiculous, that just because a boy asks you out a few times doesn't mean he has serious intentions, she still felt that the two of them had drifted apart in their aims and ideals.

Helen, though, during the last year at Salt Lake City, had subconsciously counted on Stanley to provide her with an entree into the social life of the college. While it was true that not nearly all the students paired off for the social evenings on Saturday night and for the occasional marches, it certainly was nice to have the added dimension of a male in the picture.

Oh, well, she told herself, something is bound to come along. Her optimistic nature always asserted itself at moments of discouragement. Meanwhile, there were her classes, her work, her new girlfriends, and all the rest of the college scene. The year passed on wings; summer approached. This was a new problem.

"I doubt whether I can get a job in Reno where they'll let me have Sabbath off," Helen said to her friends, remem bering her father's long struggles on that account. "And if I can't save up some money this summer, I won't be able to come back next year."

They came up with a solution. "Ask whether you can work here all summer," they told her.

Wide-eyed, Helen asked, "Do they hire students for the summer?"

Upon being informed that they indeed did, she flew to the business office, made her application, was accepted, and enjoyed the summer immensely, even with its long days of hard work. There was such a feeling of "familyness" among the students on the campus. Some of the tight restrictions were relaxed, though the essential idealism and high principles remained. The students themselves organized frequent picnics, which Helen loved. The college was full of students, actually, but they were a different breed; they were church school and academy teachers recertifying; they were mature, established people. The young students in the dormitory, Helen included, rather deplored having to remain so quiet in the evenings, after their ten-hour workdays. But the teachers had to study.

Then, without warning, a new interest developed in Helen's life. Working part-time in the business office that summer, Helen was responsible for delivering intermail all over the campus. It was never a chore; she reveled in the warm summer air. There was no such thing as a "bad" day; they were all bright and shining. On one of these bright days, when she took the mail to the store, she fell into conversation with a young man who was also working in preparation for the next year, with his bailiwick the store.

"Will you be bringing some mail again tomorrow?" he inquired, after learning her name.

"Why, yes—I come every day," Helen told him, just a bit flustered as she recognized the obvious interest in his eyes. As the weeks flew by, she and her new friend spent as much time together as possible, though not in what would be called a dating situation, since those opportunities did not exist. But they exchanged their innermost thoughts; they learned to look forward to their long, philosophical discussions. One day he said to Helen, hesitantly, "When school begins, is there any reason why our friendship can't continue?"

Helen understood what he was asking her. Was she involved romantically with anyone else? All unbidden, Stan's face drifted before her eyes. But that chapter was closed—granted that it had ever begun. This was here and now. Her new friend was a fine young man, one who shared her beliefs and convictions.

With complete sincerity, she replied, "No reason at all." His face brightened, and he beamed at her delightedly. Nothing more was said, but a great deal was understood. Helen, though, did not realize the depth of his feeling for her; she could not know that he had dreamed many dreams with her as the central figure in his future.

Then one day sad news flashed about the campus. Stan Jefferson, along with three other students, had been involved in a serious automobile accident as the four were driving in the central part of California. Banner headlines in the local newspaper screamed: "Four Youths Miraculously Escape Death." They had been hit by a soft-drink truck. Stan was seriously injured. There was a question as to his future.

On hearing this, all the old pent-up feelings rushed through Helen. She quickly excused herself and walked into the woods behind Graf Hall, where she prayed with all the earnestness of her nature that his life be spared and that the accident be a blessing, not a curse, by bringing him back to his original commitment to God. The more she prayed for him, the more he was in her mind, waking and sleeping. When he began to appear in her dreams at night, she mentally took herself by the scruff of the neck, shook herself soundly, and scolded, "Now you stop this silliness right here and now, Helen Sanford! He's forgotten you even exist."

Or had he?

She and her new friend continued to enjoy each other's company. She seemed suspended in some kind of bubble. Soon she would float down to earth and find solid footing.

It had been feared at first that Stan would not be able to return to school for his senior year because of his injuries. But when Helen caught a glimpse of him across the dining room, on crutches, his face swollen and bruised, her heart gave a great lurch. She forced herself to walk to him calmly and say, "I'm so glad that you were well enough to come back, Stan."

This time there was no mistaking it. His eyes lingered on her. He tried to prolong the brief encounter, but the hurrying students and the awkwardness of his crutches were defeating elements. But Stan would not let her go easily.

"Helen," he declared earnestly, "I want you to know that I have reconsecrated my heart to God and that I am determined to go through with my ambitions to become a minister. I know that my life was spared for a purpose."

Startled but overjoyed, Helen gazed at him speechlessly, her hyacinth eyes more eloquent than any words could have been. Stan's next words, though, were unexpected.

"I'd like to see you—to talk to you—to be with you," he told her. "Will you go with me to the banquet next week?"

Helen had thought during the preceding year that she would have given a great deal to hear those words. Yet now she hesitated. Had he really changed? Was this just a phase? Would she have another heartache if she got involved again?

"I'll—I'll let you know," she murmured, and fled, her face flushed, her eyes bright.

She felt the need of counsel. Miss Dauphinee was the obvious choice. After explaining the situation, she concluded, "I'm not sure I should be seen with him after the way he was last year."

Her wise counselor replied quietly, "This young man needs encouragement, now that he has been through such a struggle. Do you think you can help him with an attitude like that?"

Stubbornly Helen replied, "Well, maybe he ought to prove himself just a little while."

"Mr. Jefferson has so much good in him" was Miss Dauphinee's response. "I would think about it carefully, Helen."

Helen did. She also held off giving him an answer—for a day or two. Then her own strong feelings for him—she wouldn't admit that she was more than a little bit in love with him—made a negative answer impossible. Stan and Helen went to the banquet together. They both felt a sense of belonging, of having reached some destination they'd searched for a long time. And when under the tablecloth Stan's hand crept across to clasp hers for the very first time, Helen knew that what she felt for him was very special. She might never feel quite that way again. The two of them didn't need to make elaborate promises about the future. With that special sensitivity that people in love have, they took it for granted that their two fates were now going to merge.

But a note of pain and sadness interrupted the bright melody in Helen's heart when, the next day, her summer friend stopped her on the second floor of Irwin Hall. It was obvious that he was deeply hurt, deeply wounded. He had heard that she would be going to the banquet with Stan Jefferson, but hadn't been able to believe it, yet had been afraid to ask her himself, for fear it was true. Fearing rejection, he had waited through the banquet and known that his fears were all realized.

"But you told me there was no reason why our friendship couldn't continue," he reminded Helen, so obviously shattered that she was stricken with guilt and remorse. "I had made my plans around you . . ."

Helen burst into tears, her own heart aching because she had brought pain to another person. "I didn't know things would turn out this way . . . I thought my friendship with Stan was all over . . . I'm so sorry . . ."

But no words can heal these kinds of wounds. Back in her

room, she thought it over and breathed a little prayer for forgiveness and shed more and many tears for him, even though it had not been an intentional thing. As the weeks passed she heard from other students that her summer friend was really heartbroken. What a sad world this is, she said to herself. Life as it went on was kind to him, though; he later became a happy, faithful, successful doctor.

But even her sadness for another person could not dim the joy of each new day. She had found her "someday." Every morning she jumped out of bed before the rising bell rang so that she would have more time to spend on her hair. It must look just as perfect as possible—for Stan. She winnowed out a few minutes here and there to take her much-worn dresses and skirts to the pressing room so that she would always appear well-groomed—for Stan. She flew through the long hours of dictation and transcription, and her studying. Even the innocent, popular love songs of that era, with their emphasis on "forever" and idealism and faithfulness, seemed to have been written for her and Stan. She would find herself singing under her breath:

"I'll be loving you . . . always
With a love that's true . . . always.
Not for just an hour, not for just a day,
Not for just a year . . . but always . . ."

And

"Can it be the trees that fill the breeze
With rare and magic perfume?
Oh, no, it isn't the trees
It's love in bloom."

They were both so busy that spending much time together was impossible—and anyway, couples who stood about the campus talking were very apt to be called into the college president's office and severely reprimanded. So the two of them learned when they were most likely to catch glimpses of each other between classes, in chapel, in the dining room. Their eyes spoke the volumes that their tongues had no opportunity to speak. And once in a great while they arranged for a "parlor date"—that strange custom whereby a young man was allowed to call on his sweetheart in Graf Hall and spend exactly one hour in the parlor with her—with girls walking in and out, and someone usually playing the piano at top volume.

Still, in spite of the tenderness in his eyes and in his voice and in his manner when he was with Helen, he had said nothing definite. Helen's friends became curious.

"Has Stan proposed yet?" Eileen (now Helen's "fun" roommate) asked her impishly one day, herself engaged in a serious romance.

"Oh, honestly, Eileen—what a question! We don't know each other that well yet," Helen protested.

"You just wait" was Eileen's rejoinder.

Helen was willing to wait.

Then Thanksgiving vacation was coming up. Helen assumed that she might stay at the college, for it wouldn't be worthwhile to spend the money for train fare to Reno. But Eileen had other ideas. She burst into the room.

"Mother is inviting you and Stan and another couple, along with Ivan and me, to spend Thanksgiving at our house in Oakland," she told Helen. "Oh, won't we have the best time!"

Helen was almost afraid to believe this wonderful news. Four whole days with Stan with freedom to talk and to be together! Was such a thing possible? And for once, reality measured up to anticipation, for the days in Oakland, as guests in the home of Elder and Mrs. Eric B. Hare, were a time Helen never forgot. Everything was so new, so beautiful, in her relationship with Stan. And yet Stan had never even kissed her. They were so shy and so tentative with each other that their friends were amused, watching them. Finally, when the three couples went out in the little boats on Lake Merritt, Stan got his courage up; he kissed Helen, briefly and innocently, to the tune of their wildly beating hearts. But he said nothing about the future.

Then Sunday came, almost like lightning. The travel arrangements called for Eileen and Ivan to ride in the front seat with Elder Hare, with Helen and Stan in the back seat alone, the other couple having secured other transportation home. In the soft California dusk and the gathering darkness Stan put his arm around Helen, pulling her close to him. He kissed her burning cheek gently, and stroked her hands. With the feminine intuition common to women, Helen sensed that this was it. With his lips close to her ear, Stan whispered, "Sweetheart, will you be mine for life?"

Helen was in a quandary. She wanted to shout "*Yes!*" at the top of her lungs, but she didn't want the people in the front seat to hear that word. They might think—well, they might think that Stan had just proposed!

"Um hum," she murmured, her throat so tight that she could hardly manage any response at all. She never really remembered much about the rest of the ride home. She and Stan were alone in their own little world, riding on pink clouds, with heavenly music surrounding them.

But they did not really know each other at all.

Back in the dormitory, Helen confided her engagement to Miss Dauphinee, who was pleased. "You will make a wonderful minister's wife, Helen," she told the tall, willowy girl.

Helen had reservations about that, even though in her early teens she had declared that if she were lucky she might even marry a preacher! She knew that the faculty members took more interest in the ministerial couples than in any others on the campus. Very high standards were held for the girls chosen by the neophyte preachers. When a budding preacher entered denominational work, it was standard procedure to expect that his young wife would give all her time to the furthering of his calling. It was unheard of for a minister's wife to have a life or interests of her own. Moreover, she was expected to be an example both of and to the brethren in everything—dress, deportment, consecration, the ability to "make do" on a salary so slim as to be almost nonexistent. She must be outgoing, hospitable—and above all, she must play the piano well, so as to assist in her new husband's public meetings. Thinking all this over, Helen wondered whether she could measure up.

"I'll work harder than any other minister's wife ever worked," she promised herself.

Stan's parents, upon his telling them of his engagement, were understandably determined to meet his young lady at the very first opportunity. Marriage was a serious step. Had Stan chosen wisely? They insisted that Helen come to them for part of the Christmas holidays. At first she was reluctant. She saw her parents and her brothers so rarely. Surely they deserved to have her with them during the entire vacation, much as she would miss Stan. But her parents were understanding. "You are a young adult now, Helen," they told her. "It is only right that you should go to southern California and get acquainted with Elder and Mrs. Jefferson."

After she had spent a few days in Reno, Stan sent Helen money to take the train to Los Angeles. At that time Elder Jefferson was pastor of the Inglewood church. He was a minister so well-organized and so proficient at Bible studies and personal evangelism that he baptized enormous numbers of converts each year. Helen thought the parsonage the Jeffersons lived in was quite the nicest home she had ever been in. But that wasn't the thing that impressed her most.

Stan's courtesy, deference, helpfulness, and kindness to his mother and father made an indelible impression on her. She remembered what her brother Harry had said: "You should never marry a man unless you visit first in his home and see how he acts there, especially with his mother." Well, if that was the acid test, Stan passed it with flying colors. He seemed to anticipate ways to be helpful, to smooth out the rough edges. There was not a trace of condescension in his manner. (Much later on, her own mother would say, "All you need to do is think that you'd like a glass of water, and Stan gets it for you!")

The days in Stan's home were beautiful ones for Helen. She was secure and serene in her decision to marry him and to share the life he hoped to lead as a pastor-evangelist. With his lovely singing voice, she could accompany him on the piano. They were meant for each other. She thanked God over and over for bringing Stan into her life. She could not imagine wanting anything more than she now had.

Back at PUC, the glorious days of Christmas vacation faded almost immediately into the past. Money continued to be a severe problem. Her parents had never really regained any financial solidarity; her mother needed constant medical care. They had remodeled the small house into two apartments; the rent from one side of it was really all the steady income they had, between Ben Sanford's sales work. They could not help Helen with even one dollar for her schooling. Now she began working at least thirty-five hours a week as she watched her tiny bank balance begin to disappear. Often, during the second year, when she became Dr. Alvin Johnson's secretary, he would dictate at night until late; she would transcribe his letters between her classes. Sometimes she had nightmares in which shorthand notebooks full of curlicues were smothering her. She would wake up, gasping for air.

Helen continued to enter into as many aspects of college life as her work schedule permitted, full of the enormous vitality and energy she possessed. She was a familiar sight on all the long flights of steps on the campus, running at full speed, her cheeks pink, her eyes sparkling. When the English classes were invited to participate in a story contest being sponsored by *The Youth's Instructor,* at that time the periodical for young people, Helen threw herself into an article depicting her loneliness in high school and as a "working woman" when she was still so young. To her amazement and delight, she won a first prize. "Seven Years of Waiting" was published in 1938.

Both Helen and Stan were members of the a cappella choir, directed by Ivalyn Law. Helen, a natural musician, learned the difficult parts easily; Miss Law did not permit her choir members to sing with music. Stan, a recognized soloist on the campus, thrilled Helen whenever she heard him sing.

In her happy fantasies, she pictured a home with a beautiful piano or organ—parents (herself and Stan) and happy children as the whole family gathered to sing and play. How wonderful it would all be!

The time she and Stan could spend together was almost nonexistent. As the weeks passed and they became no better acquainted than during the first exciting weeks, Helen was troubled. People ought to know all about each other before they marry, she thought to herself. But there was seldom time for anything more than a hurried chat at a program or an occasional parlor date.

One thing Helen protected fiercely was time for her private devotions. Though she loved the worships Miss Dauphinee conducted each morning, still she felt a hunger for something more. She arranged her schedule so that the first period of each day was open. She resolutely refused to study her college work or to transcribe letters. In the quiet of her room, she took her Bible and the few Spirit of Prophecy books she had managed to buy over the years. She read and meditated and went out of the little room refreshed, ready to meet whatever might come.

Miss Dauphinee was apparently watching the situation carefully. She was in a novel predicament, for usually she was constantly laboring with the couples, suggesting that they not spend so much time together, that they not ask for so many parlor dates, that in general, they put the brakes on. But with Helen it was different. She could see the shadows of fatigue etching deeper each day under Helen's blue eyes, though she never complained. Miss Dauphinee pondered. Then she called Helen to her office.

"Helen," she said, "I think you really need to become a bit better acquainted with Mr. Jefferson before you marry him this coming summer. Now I certainly would not suggest this to very many of my girls, but you are a bit older, and I have unbounded confidence in you and in your friend Hedy. If you and Hedy should happen to attend church down at the St. Helena Sanitarium this coming Sabbath, and if Mr. Jefferson and Mr. Jemison should also happen to attend, and if the four of you spent the lunch hour and afternoon with Hedy's mother—I think that would be a nice plan all the way around."

Unable to believe her ears—meeting off-campus was strictly forbidden—Helen's eyes danced.

"Thank you, dear Miss Dauphinee," she beamed.

Helen never forgot the congregational song they were singing when Stan and Housel walked in: " 'A tent or a cottage, O, why should I care? They're building a palace for me over there!' " In just a few short months she'd be living with Stan in a tent, though at this moment she could not know this.

During the rare times when they were alone together, Stan was very quiet. He responded warmly to Helen's eager chatter, but at times she was troubled. Shouldn't he talk more? Shouldn't he be sharing more of his inner thoughts with her if they were going to spend their lives together? They really weren't making plans as they should. Somehow they couldn't manage to talk about things she felt they needed to discuss. She felt that Stan talked to his friends who were also headed for a life in the ministry in a frank and open way that he never talked to her. Yet there was no doubt that he loved her. Of that central fact she was absolutely sure. And she adored him with no reservations. Oh, well, she said to herself, dismissing the nagging doubts, it will all work out once we're married.

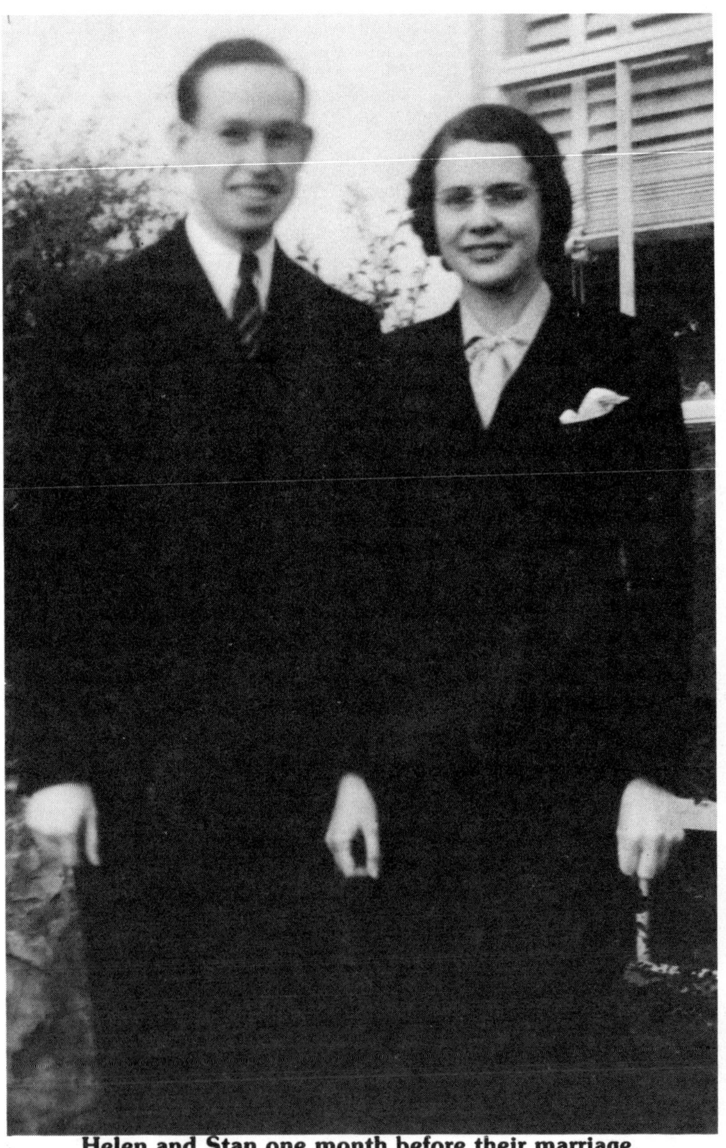

Helen and Stan one month before their marriage.

CHAPTER 7

Starting Life Together

AS THE school year drifted into spring, it began to dawn on Helen that she didn't know how in the world she could be married in June, as she and Stan had planned in one of their rare private moments together. She had few clothes and, by this time, absolutely no money. Her parents could send her only an occasional dime in a letter; a few times during the year they had managed to enclose a dollar. (At one time a dollar had come from home when her last pair of stockings were totally gone; they could not be mended further. The rules required that hose must be worn at all times. Never was a dollar more welcome.)

Miss Dauphinee was aware of her situation. "Helen," she told the blue-eyed girl earnestly, "wouldn't it be better for you to postpone your wedding for a few months and work, and save every cent so you can buy at least the most essential things to set up housekeeping?"

Helen grasped the wisdom of this suggestion at once. Moreover, she was so tired, with her work and study routine. After all, she told herself, working wouldn't be a dead-end street now that she had Stan and the prospects of their life together. Perhaps it was something they ought to think about.

When next the two of them were able to spend a few minutes together she told him of Miss Dauphinee's suggestion. He was aghast.

"But, Helen," he remonstrated, "when the Northern California Conference voted to hire me, they made it clear that my first assignment will be to hold a tent effort, either by myself or with another beginning preacher. You know they don't like to take on any fellow who doesn't have marriage prospects, so they wanted to make sure that I would be married when I started in the work. Next they questioned me carefully about whether or not you could play the piano for an effort. They said it was essential that you do this."

Seeing his consternation, Helen retreated quickly. She certainly couldn't jeopardize his entry into denominational work. After all, there weren't enough jobs to go around for all the graduating ministerial students. With the background of her experience in Salt Lake City, she knew better than to argue with conference officials.

"Well, we'll just do the best we can and manage somehow," they assured each other.

But they had no idea of what was involved or the specifics of "managing." Pacific Union College had taught them many valuable things, but it had not taught them, or any other of its students, how to be married people.

When Helen's friends learned of her uncertainty about a June wedding, they were astonished. Why, "everybody" was getting married! It was the thing to do. You went to college, you met your future husband, you married him as soon as possible, and lived happily ever after. As for money, they pointed out that an insurance settlement was bound to be made from the accident that Stan and the three others had been involved in with the truck.

"You and Stan will be rich as Croesus, while the rest of us will be dirt poor!" they announced blithely—neither "rich" nor "poor" having much meaning to them in the cocoonlike atmosphere of college.

Helen wanted to believe that this lovely future would become a reality. She wanted to marry Stan more than anything else in the world. As the days flew by, she prayed each morning during her devotions: "Lord, if there's any reason why Stan and I shouldn't marry, please show it to me. Please help us not to make a mistake. I want to do Your will in all things."

She didn't expect the Lord to send an angel down from heaven to express His will. She would use the human resources open to her, which meant questioning faculty members. Did they have confidence in Stan? They did, every one of them. Then she asked to talk to his roommate, feeling like a traitor as she did so, even the slightest intimation of disloyalty making her heartsick. But the roommate "passed" Stan with flying colors. He informed Helen that she was a lucky girl, indeed, and that there were a lot of other girls on the campus who would gladly change places with her. Hastily Helen made it clear to him that she had no doubts—she only wanted to be extra-sure.

One thing paramount in her mind was something she could do nothing about. It was her old nemesis, sickness. Helen could not shake off the horror that had been indelibly impressed on her mind at the thought of long-range sickness in a home. It was the one thing before which her faith faltered. She prayed about that, probably with more intensity than anything else. "Dear Lord, please indicate to me whether Stan or I will be an invalid—please give me a sign that we will be well," she asked the Lord.

When she wrote a long letter to her parents, explaining the situation, her mother wrote back that she felt, along with Miss Dauphinee, that Helen would be better off to work, even until Christmas.

"Helen," she wrote, "marriage is a totally different existence. You will be sharing a life space with another person, a person whom I think you do not know well, though we certainly have no objections to Stanley. Helen, you have studied and worked so hard for so long. Can't you be a little bit good to yourself just this once?"

Helen didn't see how she could, under the circumstances. It would not have occurred to her to question the fairness of a young man's employment hinging on producing a piano-playing wife.

Probably some of her insecurity stemmed from the fact

that she had grown up in Reno, Nevada, that city renowned for the quick divorce and the equally quick remarriage. As she had grown into her teens, she and her friends used to have fun checking the newspaper lists of divorces and comparing them with the lists of marriages. The same names usually appeared on both lists. The "frying pan to fire" syndrome was one she learned about early. She wanted a marriage that was forever. When she married, it was to be for keeps. Only death would dissolve the tie.

Finally, then, Helen's heart was her most effective consultant. Quite simply, her heart told her that she could not live without Stan. She did not want to live without him. He gave brightness and meaning to all her days. The old loneliness was gone, leaving in its place a feeling of being so cherished, so special, that nothing could cause her to go back. Fatigue, lack of money—even lack of real knowledge of Stan as a person—could not stop her. It boiled down to a very simple fact. She loved him unreservedly.

When Helen was sure in her own mind that her decision to marry was totally firm, she frankly confronted the necessity for securing information on the physical side of marriage. As girls have done since the beginning of time, whispers and conjectures and half-truths entered conversations—but that was the extent of her information, coupled with the negative comments poured into her ears when she was just a girl in the Reno church. (The woman separated from her husband had really left nothing to the imagination.)

Helen, the activist, approached a girlfriend whom she trusted, a girl who would be married within a few weeks of her own wedding.

"I think we ought to see a doctor," she told her friend. "We certainly need to know more than we know now—to say nothing of the fact that we absolutely *can't* have babies the first thing. Our new husbands need to get a foothold in the work before we take on babies."

"Let's make an appointment with the doctor in St.

Helena," her friend promptly suggested. "I've heard that she's a fine Christian woman."

And so Helen spent just about the last cent in her tiny bank account for her medical appointment. But she always felt that it was a bargain, for the kindly doctor spoke to her so carefully, and so frankly, and explained sexual needs and differences so clearly that she always felt her glorious happiness in her marriage was due to a great extent to her. Her girlfriend shared her feelings.

Now that was taken care of. Later on, when she and Stan were older, had established themselves, they would think about having a family.

One of the most terrifying of remarks that could be made by faculty members regarding a prospective bride was: "She'll be a hindrance to him in his work." Every fiancée of a ministerial student feared those words almost more than a death sentence. Helen had no intention of letting them be said about her. She would stand right beside her husband, shoulder to shoulder, unencumbered by a baby. It was all planned. Later she learned that Stan's father had suggested that Stan also see a doctor friend in Glendale, which he had done.

Helen was sad, though, that she would not have the lovely feminine clothes that a groom has a right to expect of his bride. "My things are so old and tired-looking," she told Eileen. "If only . . ." But there was little use in finishing the sentence.

Eileen, with her usual optimism chirped, "Everything is going to be all right, Helen, you'll see!"

Her good friend did more than encourage her verbally. About five o'clock on graduation morning Helen awakened to the sound of loud knocking on her door. What in the world? And then all her friends burst into the room, carrying a big umbrella with packages tied all around it. They sat Helen up in bed, cut one ribbon, and all the prettily wrapped packages fell on the bed with her. They had all contributed money, had sent it to Mrs. Hare in Oakland, and she had bought gowns and slips and everything else she felt Helen would need.

Her hyacinth eyes swimming with tears, Helen thanked them over and over. How lucky she was to have these wonderful friends, and Stan, and all the happy future stretching out before her. When, in a few hours, she watched Stan, in his tall young manhood, march down the aisle to receive his diploma, she had such an overflowing sense of joy that she felt her body could not contain it.

Then they parted, she and Stan, Helen to return to Reno for wedding preparations, and Stan to his parents' home in southern California, to pack his possessions and then back north to help set up tents for camp meeting in northern California at Lodi. It was now the middle of May. They would be married on June 18.

In an age before medical insurance had been thought of, a serious illness or accident could cripple a family for life, as Helen well knew. She was alarmed that many of Stan's medical bills were still outstanding, waiting on the prospect of "the settlement," two words that loomed large in the thinking of the young couple. He also had school bills unpaid, for he had not been able to work enough to keep ahead of the bills. Helen had had to sacrifice top grades to keep her bills paid; she had worked more than she had studied, but a neophyte preacher could not do this. "Well," they said to each other on the few occasions they discussed practical matters, "when the settlement comes, everything will be OK."

At home now, Helen must plan the least expensive wedding possible, in the shortest time. How she longed for a shining white satin gown—every girl's dream in that day and age. But satin was so expensive as to be completely out of the question. Browsing through the stores, examining piece after piece of white yard goods, Helen finally found a bargain bolt of white organdy. She could purchase all she would need for her wedding gown for six dollars. She wouldn't even need to make a long slip to wear under the sheer dress; Hedy, who married a few weeks before Helen, had offered her slip as well as her veil. Helen and her mother spent strained hours making the dress; then Helen managed to buy a pair of white pumps. Eileen would be her maid of honor. She would wear a dress she already owned. The groom's attendants would wear their dark, Sabbath suits. The small, simple plans were complete.

Helen and her mother found a new closeness as they planned for this vital step in Helen's life. With the sisterhood of women that marriage brings, they smiled and giggled like two contemporaries over small happenings, small incidents. And her mother made sure that Helen had the information she needed regarding the intimacies of marriage. Etta Sanford was a forthright woman.

On one thing she had had strong feelings.

"Helen, I don't want you and Stan just to answer *I do* to the preacher," she told her daughter. "Marriage is just about the most solemn thing in the world, with the most far-reaching consequences. When your father and I were married, we repeated rather long vows after the preacher, and I thought about each promise very carefully. I know he did, too. It really meant something. So I hope you and Stan will do the same."

As Helen thought it over, she felt that she also wanted to make firm and lasting promises. She knew that Stan would agree. He felt as serious as she did about marriage.

When the morning of June 18 dawned, it was hot and clear in Reno, as it always was during summer. The tiny Reno church had been scrubbed and polished. The couple had opened their few and simple wedding gifts. But as she and her father stood in the vestibule, Helen in her homemade white organdy dress, she had a sense of the glorious presence of God, confirming the commitment the two of them would make. She knew that she was making a commitment to God as well as to Stan, and in later years she would return to that commitment over and over. She would also come to believe that wedding vows can be kept only as God is taken into the marriage. In human strength it is impossible to adjust to the changing scenes of life, to continue when hope seems gone. She did not then know, mercifully, the strains, pitfalls, temptations, and tragedies that were in the future. And she did not know that as she stood there, she was beautiful—a dream bride. But Stan knew.

Leaning on her tall, solid, red-haired father, Helen prayed silently that the Lord would bless this marriage and keep it secure and happy as long as she and Stan lived.

The familiar strains of the wedding march began. Then Helen got a surprise. Just before Eileen started down the aisle, she whispered to Helen, "Stan's going to sing to you when you get to the altar!" Then Helen remembered that she and Stan had talked about this once, in one of their brief, hurried conversations, but she had thought he would be too tense, too nervous, to sing. It had never come up again. He had kept it as a surprise.

Then another beautiful surprise. Her father had arranged with one of the deacons to ring the church bells just as he and Helen started up the aisle. That tiny, white, humble church didn't have much to offer, but it did have one outstanding feature—beautiful bells. Shivers ran down Helen's back and over her entire body as the two of them, with their measured, rehearsed tread, walked down the short aisle, the melodic bells punctuating their steps. Her father paused. Stan, whose deep-brown eyes had been fixed on Helen, waited for a chord. Then he sang just to her and to her alone the beautiful old song "My Heart Is a Haven." Every word seemed written just for her, just for their love.

"When moonbeams lie shim'ring upon the waters blue
    My thoughts go a wand'ring, my dear, to you.
My dream-boats go sailing, sent forth—at love's behest,
    All laden with thoughts, dear, from one who loves you
        best.

"If wishes came true, dear, your life would be all song,
And roses be scattered your way along.
But shadows will come, love, and storms will veil the blue,
But my heart is a haven, that waits to shelter you."

Standing beside her almost-husband at the altar, Helen thought she would never again be as happy as she was in that brief, shining moment. She tried to concentrate with all her mind on the words of Elder A. H. Field, her pastor. But her emotions were almost too overwhelming. Only when it was time for the vows did all the words fall into deep and serious meaning. Then she repeated the vows unreservedly, holding back nothing: "For better or worse . . . for richer or poorer . . . in sickness and in health . . ." The last phrase stuck a tiny finger of ice at her heart. Sickness. There was that dread word again.

She and Stan repeated the vows, hands clasped, looking deeply into each other's eyes. And suddenly—they were husband and wife! Now they were going down the aisle again, this time together. Then there was the joy of the reception. Helen, who had thought to herself that her heart was so full of joy and emotion that it could not hold one drop more, found that it overflowed into rainbow tears when Stan surprised her once again at the reception. This time his song was hers alone, one he had sung to her softly during one of their few "alone" times before their wedding and one that he would sing and hum to her through the years.

"There's a little brown road windin' over the hill
To a little white cot by the sea.
There's a little green gate, by whose trellis I wait
While two eyes of blue come smilin' through—at me.

"There's a gray lock or two in the brown of your hair;
There's some silver in mine, too, I see;
But in all the long years, when the clouds brought their tears,
Those two eyes of blue kept smilin' through—at me."

I have always longed for heaven, Helen thought, her eyes starry, but now I have my own heaven here on earth. All the long years of sorrow and hard work and loneliness were gone, magically wiped out. She didn't even hear the words "clouds . . . tears"—they had no reality on this beautiful, glorious June day. She could not even think in terms of a very small dark cloud, just over the horizon, a dark cloud that would one day obscure all the brightness of her life.

Then there were flurries of congratulations, handshakes, kisses, wedding cake, punch, hugs, and then the two of them changed their clothes for their "trip" to a hotel in Reno for their wedding night.

Helen, wildly and romantically in love with Stan, had still been conscious of a feeling of apprehension as their wedding approached—not for the wedding itself, but for her wedding night. She and Stan had spent so little time together. They had never talked intimately. But she had done her best to be prepared and informed. Nonetheless, would she prove a disappointment to him? Was she ready to respond to his love?

All her fears were laid to rest. Their wedding night was a beautiful coming-together of two consecrated young Christians. Helen had not dreamed that any man could be so tender, so considerate, as Stan was. Her happiness, her satisfaction, were his only thoughts. He was infinitely gentle.

The next day, Monday morning, they packed their few gifts and Helen's few clothes into the back seat of Stan's old car and headed for Mount Lassen, in northern California, where they would spend the two or three days of their honeymoon. As they drove along, almost giddy with the newness of their shared lives, the car began to sway just a bit with the unmistakable motion prior to a flat tire.

"Oh, no!" Stan groaned. "Not a flat tire on our honeymoon. Not that."

But it was. Stan, immaculately dressed as always, got out to survey the damage, Helen close behind him. There was no way out of their dilemma but to take all the wedding gifts out of the back seat, lift out the seat, and get the jack, which was stored under the seat, as in all cars of that era. Standing beside the car, Stan and Helen laughed ruefully. Just as they were beginning the unloading of the back seat, along came a car driven by a rather strange-looking little old man in rough clothes.

"Havin' trouble?" he called.

Upon hearing of their newlywed state (who else carries wedding presents in the back seat?) he insisted on using his own jack and changing the tire, in spite of Stan's protestations.

"Shouldn't git yerself all dirty on yer honeymoon, young feller," he told him, with a wide grin.

His strange clothes looked rather like angel garments to them at that point. As they were watching the tire-change, though, with the car radio turned on, a local announcer uttered what he considered to be his joke of the day: "If love is blind, marriage is an eye-opener." Helen couldn't stop laughing. It just seemed so totally appropriate, under the circumstances.

Helen had not known that she could be so happy, that the world could be so bright and promising. Stan, who had been very restrained, very correct, during their courtship, now became warmly loving and demonstrative. He kissed Helen whenever he was near her. He patted her shoulder as he walked by. He hugged her enthusiastically at the slightest pretext. Overnight, she became "Snooksie, Dolly-babe, Precious One." Every scar of loneliness that she had carried in her lifetime was erased. Helen was almost afraid of her happiness; it was so boundless, so all-encompassing. Did human beings truly have a right to be this happy? As they went boating on the lake, Helen even choked down her fear of drowning. Stan was total security.

This tiny moment in the time frame of their lives passed with lightning speed. They had to push on to the little town of

Mount Shasta, in northern California, where Stan would preach his maiden sermon on Sabbath. They had to get settled so the effort they were to hold could be started. It would all be marvelous, though, for they had learned that Hedy and Housel, themselves just married, would join them for the effort.

"We have to look for a tiny house or an apartment to rent the first thing, so we can organize ourselves for the meetings," Helen told Stan.

He gulped. "Didn't I tell you—how could I have forgotten—that we'll be living in a tent next to the big tent——"

Seeing Helen's blue eyes open wide, he hurried on. "But Housel and Hedy will be living in one just like it, and we'll have a lot of fun together."

At this point nothing—certainly not the prospect of living in a tent—could have dimmed Helen's happiness. And she and Stan and the Jemisons had such fun that never would they forget it as the years rolled along. Mrs. Elkins (known as Mother Elkins) took in the four of them until the tents were ready, cooked the most amazing quantities of good food, and in general became like a member of both families. Helen and Hedy chided their new husbands about eating so much.

"Well, we certainly can't let it go to waste," they replied happily. "And besides, who knows? These may be the last good meals we'll ever get!"

But the brides were resolved that this would not be the case.

Helen and Hedy stood on the sidelines and cheered as their new husbands wrestled with the intricacies of tent-pitching, a skill that was not taught in their training for the ministry.

"We're going to make these tents just like palaces for you girls," the grooms boasted. "Why, you'll never want to leave them!"

The girls smiled indulgently at each other. The boys went

to a mill, purchased a quantity of knotty pine, built floors, and installed them. Then they built a privacy fence around the two tents. Down the middle of each tent they ran a partition, with built-in closets on one side. They also made "kitchen shelves" at the back. Helen, getting into the spirit of the thing, shopped at the dime store for red-and-white-checked gingham for curtains, which she sewed by hand, to keep the dust off her dishes. There was even a padlock so that the closet containing their few valuable possessions could be locked when they were away from the tent.

"Stan," Helen exclaimed, as the tents were taking shape, "do you realize we don't even have a bed? We've been staying with church members—I completely forgot that we don't own a stick of furniture."

Stanley agreed that this was a problem indeed. Hedy, though, had worked as secretary to the president of the conference. She knew a number of the laity; she also had learned how to get things done. To their great joy, she managed to get them a bed. Now, with two folding chairs, and a knotty-pine table the two boys built, they were almost living in "style." Their other items of furniture consisted of Helen's unfinished cedar chest. Housel, interested in fine woodworking, had built a cedar chest for Hedy that last year of college. In a burst of happy generosity, he'd offered to build one for Helen, with Stan buying the materials. Unfortunately, with the pressure of graduation, he hadn't finished it. So there it sat—but at least it could be used for storage.

"What will we do about water?" was the girls' next question. It was all well and good to hook up two little hot plates, and to cover a length of board with oilcloth, and to hang a mirror on the middle partition, but what about water?

"Just wait," they were told. On their next foray into town the young preachers got two fifty-gallon metal barrels from a bakery. In these they proceeded to cut and solder faucets. When the tanks were placed on wooden blocks in each tent, the inventors stood back and beamed.

"We'll fill the tanks the first thing each morning," the brides were informed. "That way, you'll always have 'running' water." And they did—after a fashion. But the running was usually so slow that in their haste the girls got into the habit of dipping into the tanks with a clean pan.

With problems being solved one by one, there remained the question of how they would bathe. Helen remembered her sponge-bath days in Salt Lake City; she hadn't anticipated retrogressing to that point again. But there were no big galvanized tubs to be bought in the little town of Mount Shasta; the country was gearing up for World War II. Metals were in short supply. All right, "spit baths" it would be—though later they did secure a very shallow, very wide tub, which was never Helen's pride and joy.

Then the more embarrassing problem of a toilet had to be taken care of. Stan had dreaded telling Helen that he had been told by the conference officials to "make arrangements to use the toilets at the closest gas station. Offer the attendant a small sum of money," they had said. Noticing his stricken silence, they had told him, "All the couples living in evangelistic tents do this."

This meant, for Helen and Hedy, a walk of about half a block, then crossing the main highway, dodging in and out of traffic. Often the restroom would be in use by motorists buying gas and they would have to stand in the hot sun, or later, in pouring rain and wind. It became obvious that this was not a practical solution for the dark hours of the night. So the newlyweds stifled their embarrassment and bought chamber pots, though Helen could hardly bear to use theirs—everything was so public.

For that matter, the total lack of privacy was a difficult blow for Helen to surmount. In some ways, she and Stan were still almost strangers; they needed time to grow into the comfort and intimacy that makes marriage so special. But there was no time for this, no opportunity. There were handbills to prepare, music to rehearse, and as the meetings progressed and Stan began to do more of the speaking, sermons to prepare. Then almost immediately there was constant visiting to do, as people signed cards at the meetings, indicating their interest. And the daily routines of life were doubly—or more—hard in a tent. Stan had come from a family who had camped for recreation. Helen had not, except for her brief stint as a junior camp counselor. Food could not be preserved for any length of time. It must be bought almost from meal to meal. The laundry was done in an old machine at Mother Elkins'.

But when she was playing the piano for the meetings, with Stan leading the music, and later, when she played for his solo each night, such a feeling of love and tenderness swept over her that tent living was the least of her worries. They had found each other, or, more precisely, now had an opportunity to find each other, emotionally and psychologically.

Each morning Stan and Helen shared a tender moment. From the first day of their married life he had instituted a unique custom. He always took her watch, wound it, and slipped it on her wrist, always accompanying the ritual with a warm, loving kiss on her hand. At those times Helen felt as though she were the most fortunate woman on earth. She felt unworthy of so rich and expressive a love as Stan's.

Then a totally unplanned-for event took place. Suddenly, after two months, Helen was becoming very nauseated in the mornings. She vomited violently. The weather was turning cold. It was autumn. She was pregnant.

For both Helen and Stan the blow was almost too much to be borne. They had absolutely no money; Stan's salary was fifteen dollars per week, and he still owed medical and school bills. "The settlement" had not come. It was of vital importance for him to establish a foothold in denominational work. In that day and age, neophyte preachers were pitted against one another in a strongly competitive way. It was made very clear to them that if they did not produce, they would be dismissed and their places given to someone more worthy. A wife was a vital factor in the early success or failure of the new preacher.

Helen felt that she had failed Stan utterly. She flung herself across their bed, sobbing. "How could this have happened? How?" she cried over and over. "You may never get to be a preacher. And it's all my fault."

As he smoothed her hair and kissed her, he asked, "How could it be all *your* fault? Snooksie, you're a big girl. You know better than that." And he would try to make her smile.

But she would not be comforted. "How can we be good parents when we don't even *want* a baby?" she wept. "Babies should be wanted!"

Gently he answered, "Then we must ask the Lord to help us want the baby."

In later life, Helen would often think over those young days when she felt so trapped and full of panic. Would their lives have been different if they could have had four or five years without children? If they could have established their own relationship more fully, and gotten a financial foothold, would life have been so hard subsequently? Stan tried in every way to be as kind as possible to Helen, but he was young and inexperienced. A baby was the last item on his list of priorities at that time of his life, when he was just blossoming into manhood.

As soon as Helen and Stan knew without a shadow of a doubt that they would be parents, they sat down to figure out what they would do financially. Medical insurance had not yet been thought of. The conferences did not provide medical benefits. Stan, by careful inquiry, found that it would cost sixty dollars for the baby to be born at the St. Helena Sanitarium, seven miles down the hill from Pacific Union College. Marvin and his wife now lived at PUC. It seemed best for Helen to plan to go there, in an age when after delivery a mother was kept in bed in the hospital for ten days, and spent more time at home in bed upon being discharged. The sixty dollars included the doctor's fee, the anesthetic—everything. But it might as well have been six thousand. They did not have even one dollar.

"We have to save five dollars a month," Helen declared. Later, after the first shock had worn off, she told Stan, "I must have been stupid when I said we had to save five dollars. We have to save more than that in order to have the sixty dollars by the time the baby comes."

There was nothing to do but eat only the barest minimum of plain food and put every penny aside. That was how they saved—in pennies. There was no money for maternity clothes for Helen. She would have to get by somehow with a dress or two given her by her sister-in-law. Prenatal care? A local doctor supplied it free to a "minister." Otherwise, they could not have afforded it. Then, as the weather worsened and the tent meetings were over, Stan was almost desperate. He felt that Helen, pregnant and sick, could not continue to live in the cold tent. He explored every inch of the little town of Mount Shasta. His persistence was rewarded with a little apartment, half-finished.

"I'll help finish up all the work here if you'll just let us move in now," he told the landlady, who knew a bargain when she saw one. It was now October; in this high altitude their water was frozen in the "tank" each morning. And, sick as she was, Helen had to take the walk across the highway to the toilet. The little apartment, with its knotty-pine walls, seemed like the anteroom of heaven. Later, though, lying in bed nauseated to the point of cold sweat, the knotty-pine whorls seemed to intensify her discomfort. She developed a lifelong aversion to knotty pine.

CHAPTER 8
A Foothold in the Ministry

IF THEY learned nothing else during these early days of their youth and inexperience, Stan and Helen learned to live by faith. They learned the practical aspect of simply taking their great need to God and placing it in His hands. For instance, there was the matter of the "Rock Crusher."

When Stan went back home after graduation to get ready for marriage and the ministry, he was without a car. A new car was as far out of reach as an ocean liner. He and his father spent days tirelessly exploring all the used-car lots in the area of Greater Los Angeles where the Jeffersons were located. The used cars with the smallest price tags seemed completely disreputable. Finally they found a used DeSoto, a much-praised car of that era. If nothing else, this vehicle would provide riding comfort; it would also be roomy enough to transport the passengers Stan was sure to have as a young preacher. He bought it.

Helen and Stan were used to the fearful noise this vehicle made. But when Hedy and Housel first encountered its rattles and squeals, they burst out laughing. "What in the world is that?" they demanded. They promptly dubbed it "The Rock Crusher," a name it retained throughout the months Helen and Stan owned it. Finally it simply expired—leaving Stan in a terrible dilemma. In that part of California in that age, a young preacher couldn't *be* a young preacher without a car. Stan had a Sabbath preaching appointment at the extreme edge of the large district. It was Thursday when the car breathed its last. A friendly mechanic gave Stan the bad news that repairs would cost more than the car itself. In their distress, they turned to God. They explained their great need. "We're trying to share the good news of Thy love with others," they told Him. "Please provide a way." Their prayer was answered. Almost miraculously a 1936 Chevrolet became available, a car that would have been totally outside their financial reach had it not been for one circumstance. An epidemic of infantile paralysis had California in its grip. People were terrified at the very words. The forest ranger, whose personal car it was, had just died of the dread disease. His wife, grief-stricken, owned a car of her own. She was selling everything she could, preparatory to moving away. The car had only 16,000 miles on it, since the ranger had used a State car for all his work. Now his widow would let the Chevrolet go for only $350. But there were no buyers. The townspeople were sure that polio germs were everywhere in the car. But the widow explained to Stan that her husband had not even been near the car for weeks before his death. He could not possibly have "infected" it. Stan needed to hear no more. With a sympathetic bank, he arranged for the lowest possible monthly payments, the mechanic bought the old "Rock Crusher" for a minimum amount, and Stan and Helen reveled in their first passable possession.

An unexpected ramification of the new car purchase was that the elderly ladies Helen and Stan had transported to all the church and tent-effort meetings now refused to ride in the "infected" car. Though the young couple wouldn't have gotten rid of their passengers voluntarily, they did enjoy the few extra minutes of private time together their car errands provided.

And so the months flew, and now in a few weeks their first baby would arrive. By now Stan and Helen were full of anticipation. They were going to be *parents*! They were finally grown up, fully and completely. Helen's mother was concerned; her little girl was going to become a mother. She would need some help. Kind church members had given Helen a simple baby shower. With the few things she had, and her undefeated spirit ("If you can't get it for yourself, don't ask; do without"), she would manage. But logistics had to be considered. Finally, it was arranged; about a month before her "due" date, Helen would go to Marvin and Eleanor at Pacific Union College.

On the ride from Mount Shasta to PUC, Helen's heart was heavy. And she felt almost disoriented. This was the college she had so loved. She remembered arriving only a few years before, full of eager plans when everything was ahead. She had left here only a little more than a year ago. So much had happened. Was this really she—heavy, swollen—sitting beside her handsome young husband? Stealing a glance at him, she realized that he looked tired, weary. Dear, dear Stan. He was working so hard. He gave everything he had to his ministry. He really didn't need a baby just yet. But mentally she shook herself. That was a road leading nowhere. But how she hated to see him turn the car in the direction from which they'd come, after he had unloaded her things. She hugged him fiercely.

"I'll let you know the very moment I start into labor," she told him.

He whispered back, "I'll be praying many times a day that everything will go well."

She'd tried to get him to say, time and again, whether he preferred a boy or a girl, but he wouldn't choose. "A healthy, happy baby, Snooksie," he told her.

Stan missed her greatly, as she missed him. Phone calls were much too expensive—and besides, Marvin and Eleanor didn't have a phone. Helen and Stan kept the mailman busy. He, dignified and composed in public, was totally articulate in writing. On May 7, 1940, he wrote:

> Darling,
>
> Today has been the longest day of my history. I have had to study all day, which has almost been an impossibility. I can hardly think of anything but you, sweetheart. I think I'd die of lonesomeness if I had to spend many days like this without you.

> I must confess that I have even shed a few tears over the matter! I just guess I must love you.
>
> The train was derailed someplace down the line this morning, so the mail didn't get here until this afternoon. I was glad to get your card and letter. You're the sweetheart when it comes to letter-writing—I would make a good ditch digger when it comes to writing letters. It's easy to write to you, though. I don't have to stop and think like I do when I write to someone else. I just love you so that all I have to do is tell you so. And you're so much in love with me that you don't know whether or not it's a good letter!
>
> Glad that you got the maidenhair ferns. Be very careful, though, when you are hiking around, that you don't trip and fall. I know you will. I pray for you every day—that the Lord will keep His protecting arm around you, 'cause you're mine, and I love you and couldn't live without you.

And then a signature too private to be shared with anyone else. He had used his typewriter to construct a line of hugs and kisses with the universal "X" and "O" symbols.

While she waited for the baby he wrote nearly every day, with such love and such reassurance that much of her first-baby fear left her. Big and pregnant as she was, he made her feel like his light-footed, willowy sweetheart again. For one letter, he cut out a heart and colored it pale pink, pasting a "Gerber baby" picture both inside and out. And this time he concluded his letter, "Tell Dougie that his daddy loves him, too, but not as much as he loves his little sweetie pie."

The two of them had gotten into the habit of referring to the baby as "Dougie," in honor of Stan's former roommate, Doug Marchus. They fell into the same pattern with Helen's second pregnancy, but the name never proved prophetic.

Early one morning Helen called Eleanor into the room. "I'd better go to the hospital right away," she gasped, frightened by the great event that was taking place with no volition on her part.

Her sister-in-law smiled indulgently. "Listen, Helen. A first baby takes an awfully long time to arrive. Now just settle down and be patient. Why, it might even be a couple of days! But if it will make you feel any better, take your watch and time the pains."

Hanging onto the doorknob for support, Helen discovered that the pains were coming almost one on top of another. Again she called. This time, after examining her briefly, Eleanor turned white and ran from the room. It had been arranged that they would borrow the landlord's car; Marvin (a student) and his wife did not own one. Her sister-in-law saw a friend passing by.

"Go and get Marvin at the post office where he works and tell him to get here as fast as he can!" she cried. "We have to get Helen down to the hospital as soon as possible."

Breathlessly she phoned Stan from the neighbor's house. Marvin arrived, and they raced down the winding road, Helen having to stifle her moans as the pains washed over her again and again. When they took her into the hospital, the nurse took one look, got her on a stretcher, and went flying with her through the old porches that used to connect one building with another at the St. Helena Sanitarium.

Meanwhile, Stan, in a fever of impatience, had to conduct an early-morning temperance committee meeting. He didn't know how to cancel the meeting, though in later years he would wish that he had. Helen, in the delivery room, yearned for Stan. If only he were here at this moment when she needed him most. If only . . . By the time he did arrive, he was already the father of a red-haired baby girl, as an acquaintance announced to him when he entered the hospital. He breathed a great sigh of relief. And when he stood by Helen's bed, and saw those blue, blue eyes so full of joy, he felt a lump in his throat. All the way in the car he had prayed that Helen would have an easy time. No prayer was ever more generously answered. Surely few first babies enter the world with as little difficulty as did Jacquee (Jacquelin)—in only three hours.

After a few weeks they were back in Mount Shasta. Now

they were three. Now their sleep was interrupted by a tiny red-haired baby who seemed to be a confirmed nocturnal creature. Now Stan's small salary must stretch around milk and baby food, medical attention for the baby, and baby clothes.

When sometimes they would become downcast and life seemed endlessly grim, they had one "magic" letter they took out and read over. Stan had sent the check for Helen's hospital expenses to the St. Helena Sanitarium in April, with the baby not due until June. His former dean of men, Walter B. Clark, now assistant manager of the hospital, was so impressed that he wrote back with the receipt at once.

April 9, 1940

Mr. Stanley Jefferson
Mt. Shasta, California

Dear Stanley:

Surprises may be the order of the day but I want to tell you this is a new one. I wish you could inject the idea into some more of our good friends to pay for service in advance. It strikes me just right. You will find enclosed our receipt in response to your remittance, and I want you to know that we do very much appreciate it.

We will be glad to do everything we can to be of assistance, and we pray for both of you Heaven's richest blessing.

I look back with more than usual pleasure on my contact with you in the dormitory. I know that the Lord has been good to you, and I am so thankful that you are finding your place in His work.

Your sincere friend,

W. B. Clark, Assistant Manager
St. Helena Sanitarium & Hospital

"Dearest," Helen told her young husband, "there's no doubt in my mind that you could be Secretary of the Treasury of the United States if you set your mind to it!"

Flattered and pleased, he replied with mock loftiness, "Well, I have much more important things to do here!"

Financial problems, though, were always there, like an ice cube in the pit of the stomach. Proud as they were, the two of them would not ask for help from their parents. "If you can't get it for yourself, do without it!" But kindly church members were aware of their struggles. In the aftermath of the depression, people tended to look out for one another. Mother Elkins, in particular, made a habit of bringing bags of food to the young couple, presenting them so tactfully and so unobtrusively that there was no humiliation involved. How grateful they were!

When one day she happened in while Helen was patching Stan's "best" white shirt, she said nothing. But later that day she brought a package.

"Now this is something I want Brother Jefferson to have," she told Helen firmly. "I'm so happy to be able to do this; I consider it a privilege to help two of God's young workers during this hard time." It was a new white shirt.

Dear Sister Elkins. They never forgot her.

However strong their optimism, finances continued to be a continual, anguishing problem. During the first year they had assured each other again and again that "when the settlement is made . . ." Everything hinged on that settlement. It had been their star of hope.

When, one quiet day, the envelope arrived from the lawyer, they were afraid to open it. They hugged their anticipation to themselves. At last, at last, the hardest days would be over! They could pay for their car. They could have some simple furniture instead of the crates and folding chairs with which they made do. They could buy a few clothes—particularly a new dark suit for Stan, who must be dressed properly every night and every Sabbath. Why, there was no end to what they would do.

Stan opened the envelope. He glanced at the check. His face turned so pale that Helen was alarmed.

"How much is it?" Helen gasped.

"It's only—it's only—why, it's just barely enough to clear

off my college bill and the doctor bills from the accident," he whispered unbelievingly.

"But that's not possible!" Helen cried. "We've counted on it! We have to have some money, or we can't go on. Everyone told us we'd be getting such a lot! What will we do—"

She broke off, suddenly realizing that Stan, in his quiet way, had counted on the money far more than she had. With a lightning flash of perception, she realized he was cut to the quick by his inability to provide better for her and the baby.

"Don't worry, sweetheart," she told him, hugging him fiercely. "We'll manage. I've never had any money in my whole life, and there's no point in breaking the pattern," she cajoled, trying to cheer him. But his face retained that bleak, drained look.

Through her happiness since her marriage, Helen had at times been conscious of a small spot of uneasiness that she always tried to ignore. Stan seemed to say so little. He communicated so briefly with her, except in letters. Always he responded to her cheerful chatter; always he was loving and kind. But she often had the feeling that he was remote, that he was living in a land alien to her. If only she knew what he was thinking! She didn't want to be a nagging wife. Sometimes when she heard the sound of her own voice, she was afraid that perhaps she had already drifted into that fault. And so the two of them, loving each other, had not really "found" each other.

Helen had discovered, early in her marriage, that when she displeased Stan, he would retreat into an icy silence that might last for days, speaking only the barest minimum of words to keep the mechanics of their lives running. Impulsive and outgoing herself, quick to speak and quick to repent, she found his unbendingness such a torture that she bent over backward to avoid these episodes. Yet it was not always possible to think ahead of her tongue.

Once her mother had said to her, "Helen, why don't you

say something once, then let it go, instead of repeating it and repeating it?"

Shocked, Helen had thought it over. The picture it created was that of a shrewish, nagging wife, the last thing in the world she wanted to be. She wondered whether her own conduct caused some of Stan's remoteness. She resolved to do better.

Helen had also learned that tears were an ineffective way of dealing with conflicts between herself and Stan. Somehow, tears antagonized him, turned him cold and unfeeling. She tried, as the years went on, to choke them back. But many times she did not succeed. And many times Stan's apparent callousness in these situations wounded her.

But another worry had not materialized. When she became pregnant, she had sometimes told herself that becoming a parent physically is a relatively simple matter. But how does a man become a father psychologically? A woman carried a child in her very body; it was already part of her being when it was born. Would Stan feel "fatherly"? She needn't have worried. Finances, tears, and other problems might arise, but there was never a problem with his love for the baby.

Helen loved to hear Stan give Bible studies during this period of their lives. He had such a gentle, quiet way of presenting the great truths. He was a personal worker of a very high quality indeed. But she sympathized with the problems he faced in preparing sermons. After the Jemisons were sent to another part of the conference and Stan preached regularly, he studied early and late. The young ministers of that era did not have the advanced training that would later become available. Lacking money, they could not buy a library. They must depend on the Bible and on the few Spirit of Prophecy books they owned. It was sink or swim, every single sermon.

When the Jeffersons were sent to another small town, Stan felt that Helen had washed by hand long enough, especially since she had so few baby clothes that daily washing was a necessity. She found an old wringer washer for fifteen dollars. It got a real workout when the other two couples in the effort found they had no place to wash. Helen invited the two other wives to wash at her house, assigning each of them a day. But the water had to be heated on the stove; the house became an inferno each washday. Little Jacquee, restless and irritable, cried nonstop.

Helen was concerned that the baby didn't seem to be growing as rapidly as she should. She was concerned about her own lack of energy and Stan's never-rugged constitution. She wondered whether her strength of old would ever return. Unable to buy high-quality, nourishing foods, the two of them settled for an impoverished diet high in sweets and carbohydrates.

When Jacquee was in the process of outgrowing her bassinet, Helen hesitantly mentioned it to Stan. "What will we do?" she asked. "How can we buy a crib?"

He passed his hand wearily across his eyes. "Let's pray about it, Snooksie," he told her. And they did. And just as miraculously as the car had appeared, a neighbor dropped in to say that another neighbor nearby had left a beautiful crib in their house when they moved out. "They wondered whether you knew of anyone who could use it," they said. They certainly did! Rushing to the empty house, they found a lovely crib, solidly paneled, with attractive wood scallops around the top. They stepped out in faith and bought a clean new mattress for Jacquee. And they didn't forget to thank their heavenly Father for anticipating their needs even before they asked.

Now Stan called Helen "Precious Little Mommy" as often as "Snooksie," his voice full of such overwhelming tenderness that Helen felt like the richest woman on earth. Their family worships were filled with love for God and for each other and for their little red-haired girl. In spite of the everyday stresses, both young people were growing in grace;

they were growing in knowledge of each other; they were learning to bring others into a new life. Somehow neither of them made a direct connection between their lack of money and Stan's occupation. Being in the ministry was the greatest privilege that a man could have. Money was unrelated to that.

There was, however, a nagging problem, one that had existed from the first days of their marriage. It had become intensified by parenthood. Helen found that if she disagreed with Stan as to how Jacquee should be disciplined and trained, she was subjected ever more frequently to his icy silences.

"It's not fair!" she told herself one day, during an episode of this sort. "He can't be right *all* the time. I'm right *some* of the time!"

But she couldn't live without his tenderness and approval. Surely sacrificing her own opinion from time to time was a small price to pay.

Next stop—Yuba City, another small town in northern California, where Stan would work with Elder Wilton Lockwood. Helen told Stan, "I heard somewhere that three moves is as hard on furniture as a fire."

"Then we can be thankful we didn't have anything of value to begin with!" he replied.

But the constant packing and unpacking and meeting new churches and gaining the confidence of the members was not an easy assignment. After a brief stay in a house borrowed from a church member—a house so dirty that Helen gagged as she tried to clean the toilet—they managed to find a small bungalow in a little court of houses at the edge of town. The houses were so small that it was impossible to wash in them. A washhouse for the court was at the other end of the row. Now, in the biting wind and rain of winter, Helen had to bundle Jacquee up and take her, along with the soiled clothes, to the warehouse, where it was cold, moist, and drafty. But the baby could not be left alone in the house where Helen could not even hear her cry. Stan was always out, tirelessly visiting the new members, passing out handbills, giving Bible studies, and in general keeping things going—or he was studying for his sermons.

One day, though, noticing the circles under Helen's eyes, he said cheerfully, "Precious Little Mommy, why don't you give me the things that have to be washed and I'll go down to the washhouse and do them—and you can stay here and transpose this song that I'm going to sing at the meeting tonight. I've been studying all morning. The change will do me good."

Helen's musicianship had suffered by not having a piano for practice. She no longer felt that she could transpose at sight. Thankfully she agreed to his suggestion. Now she and Jacquee settled down, Helen hard at work writing out the music. Then came a knock at the door. A woman church member pushed her way inside and demanded, "Where is Brother Jefferson?"

Helen, confused and startled, stammered, "Why—why—he's down at the washhouse, doing the baby's laundry."

The woman exclaimed in outrage, "Why, I never heard of such a thing! The washing is your job! What in the world—"

And before Helen could explain, before she could tell the woman that she and Stan were up until midnight every night studying and preparing music and that Helen had to take Jacquee along to the meeting every night, so that she couldn't accomplish anything except in the daytime when Jacquee was asleep, and that more than anything in the world she was dedicated to her husband's success—the woman had huffed off.

When Stanley brought back the wet clothes, he found Helen in tears. "I'm going to be a hindrance to you," she wept on his shoulder. "I know it. I'm not doing my share."

Stan wouldn't even listen to that. "Snooksie, you do so

much more than your share," he told her tenderly. "Just forget this whole thing."

But they didn't have a chance to forget it, for the woman appointed herself a committee of one to settle matters for the young Jeffersons. She went to the conference office and asked for an appointment with the administrators there. "Brother and Sister Jefferson don't belong in the ministry," she told them. "They're both lazy, and she's the worst, expecting him to do the washing!"

When the administrators, who promised to investigate, brought up the matter, Helen was terrified. "They may dismiss you from the ministry," she told Stan, as her knees weakened under her.

"They certainly wouldn't be that unfair," he replied. And he was right. He and Helen were given gentle counsel, nothing else. But never again would she let Stan help her with tasks considered strictly female, no matter how overworked she was, and no matter how much time she spent on his work.

As Jacquee grew and became a full-fledged member of the family, Helen and Stan gave thanks to God many times for having answered their prayers for a healthy, happy baby and for having planted overwhelming love in their hearts for her. Helen found herself lingering most often in the children's department of local stores, looking at the pretty little dresses, nightgowns, coats, and hats. If only she could afford to buy the beautiful clothes for her baby that some women took so for granted! When she and Stan attended the General Conference session held in San Francisco, their way financed by the conference, Helen was puzzled as to how she would manage clothes for Jacquee.

"It's always cold in San Francisco," she told Stan. "At night the fog and wind can really bite into you."

Suddenly she thought of an old white suit that she had worn until it was threadbare. She took it apart and carefully pressed all the pieces. Then she cut out a little coat, sewing all of it by hand and pressing it over and over so that the many "pieced" areas would be less noticeable. But it really wasn't warm enough for San Francisco.

When the three of them met Stan's parents in San Francisco, the latter took one look at the lovely red-haired baby girl, then took her downtown and bought a beautiful aqua wool coat and hat for her. Helen never forgot that coat and hat.

One aspect of parenthood that Helen and Stan hadn't counted on was Jacquee's energy and hand-waving, the little hands managing to connect with their glasses and shattering them on the sidewalk time and again. With no financial help for medical bills, and their bare budget, these events were always major crises. Yet somehow they couldn't manage to stay out of the range of those happy little hands.

"Snooksie," Stan said one day, "we've got to figure out a way to get food other than buying or stealing it!"

She giggled along with him, a vision going through her mind of the two of them—preacher and wife—rushing into a grocery store, grabbing all they could from the shelves, then fleeing!

"I can't see why the Bible custom of 'gleaning' couldn't be used today," he mused aloud. "I could make arrangements with orchard owners——"

"And when peaches are in season, we could pick those off the ground, and we could go through berry vines after the pickers have been through—and how about walnuts—" Helen interrupted, getting into the spirit of the thing.

Suiting the word to the deed, Stan wasted no time in making his arrangements. The fresh produce provided a greatly needed variety in their diet. They made a game of thinking up innovative ideas for securing food without cost. One day, though, as they were sitting at the dinner table, Helen suddenly announced, "I've eaten so many wild mustard greens I hope I never see them again!" (In later years, she couldn't even swallow them.)

Just about this time Stan found a cut-rate grocery store where they went once a week. They were able to buy two sacks of groceries at one dollar each. They carefully examined the dented cans, bent cereal boxes, and cartons of eggs with one or two slightly cracked. Somehow they were managing.

Then Helen faced some new challenges in the culinary department. She and Stan had invited his parents to visit them in their northern California location after the General Conference session in San Francisco. Helen had looked over her food supplies. She had made list after list of menus. With what she had canned and gleaned and the few fresh things she would need to buy, such as milk, she could produce good meals, she thought, for the duration of the visit.

Everything went beautifully until the last dinner. This was the time when frozen foods had just been introduced to the market; in fact, frozen peas were the only article available. Everyone was excited by this unbelievable delicacy, now available the year around. Suddenly Stan's mother had an inspiration. "Stan, why don't you go to the store and buy a package of frozen peas for dinner?" she exclaimed. A rather large package was priced at only twenty-five cents. But it might as well have been twenty-five dollars at that point as far as Stan and Helen were concerned.

There was a moment of silence. Helen, realizing Stan's embarrassment, spoke. "Mother Jefferson, Stan has no money at all."

Mrs. Jefferson was sorry she had suggested the peas; she hadn't realized that the young people were in quite such straits. Opening her purse, she handed Stan a dollar. "Here," she said, "this will be my treat."

When Stan returned home with the peas, he carefully handed her the seventy-five cents. Helen noticed that her mother-in-law dropped the change into one of the teacups in the cupboard, a circumstance that became woven into her next challenge.

That night Elder H. M. S. Richards, speaker for the Voice of Prophecy, and his quartet, the King's Heralds, were to hold a meeting in the town, and they had been assigned to sleep in the very large, partly furnished house in which Helen and Stan were occupying a few rooms. Helen, as the young minister's wife, was told at the last minute the group would have breakfast at her home. But nothing was said about financial arrangements. Moreover, she was due at the meeting to take care of her own duties there.

Panic overwhelmed her. What could she do? Suddenly she remembered the seventy-five cents her mother-in-law had left in the teacup. Dressing hurriedly for the meeting, she said to Stan, "I'll get up very early in the morning and rush to that little grocery store that opens so early. I can buy enough milk and a few eggs and a loaf of bread. Then with the canned fruit and fresh fruit you just picked, we can have a good breakfast."

After the night meeting, Elder Richards stopped and brought home ice cream for the crowd. He could not know what a rare treat it was for the young Jeffersons.

"We have some nice fresh blackberries," Helen twinkled. "We can have blackberry sundaes." (Blessed be Stan's berry-gleaning!) They all fell upon the sundaes with enthusiasm. As they ate, Elder Richards regaled them with stories of his own sacrificial life in the ministry. "I don't know what I would have done without the courage of my wife," he declared. "Every time we really had to have something, like a suit of clothes for me, we prayed, and the Lord provided it!"

Helen, listening appreciatively, couldn't afford to let her eyes meet Stan's lest the two of them be unable to contain themselves. To herself she was saying, "Oh, Elder Richards, if you only knew!"

Years later, she would look back on this incident and others like it and realize that the most prudent solution would have been to confess her predicament to some of the church members. They would have been more than willing to bring in food or help her out in any way they could. But she was strongly indoctrinated by the philosophy taught her at home; she also was all too keenly aware of the prevailing theory that if a young couple couldn't cope, they probably weren't meant for the ministry. She was afraid that if she asked for help, she might, in a very real sense, be jeopardizing Stan's future. When one is young, sometimes his understandings are not complete.

But soon it was time to move again—this time to Mendocino, on the coast. At first Helen had been overjoyed, for plans were laid for the Jemisons to work again with the Jeffersons. They would be living in one of the most beautiful parts of California. But alas for their dreams! A quick decision at the conference office sent the Jemisons to another area. Helen and Stan could find only one vacant house to move into, a house that rented for (to them) the astronomical sum of twenty-five dollars per month. With their check being only $125, this was indeed a large rent. They were coping with food, clothes for three, car payments, tithe, offerings, medical expenses, gasoline—to list just a few items. Feeling that she was being generous, the landlady offered to have the entire house repainted and put into excellent shape if only they would agree to pay thirty dollars. But the two of them were appalled. The Lord was coming soon. They had no right to waste money. Every cent should be put into warning the world of impending doom. The outbreak of World War II—Pearl Harbor and the rest—made the need for economy more imperative.

"Stan, how in the world will we keep the baby warm in this cold, misty climate with this green, wet redwood?" Helen wailed, trying to start a fire in the house's one stove. They learned, when they consulted "natives" about the intricacies of burning redwood, that the latter must be left outdoors a couple of seasons for the rain to wash the acid from the wood, otherwise it would simply smoke and smolder. But all the seasoned wood was gone; only "green" was available.

With a washing to do every day (Jacquee still had a decidedly limited wardrobe) Helen burst into tears of frustration when time after time the fire went out and the water on the stove stayed merely tepid.

"I've had enough," Stan declared. "I'm going to borrow a trailer and drive to the lumberyard in Willits, where I know the manager. I think he'll let me have some pine." The plan worked out—except that the pine was also green and wet!

Almost immediately after they had moved in, Helen began to itch. Then she noticed large red swellings all over her body. It seemed to her that she was on fire from head to foot. But surely she would recover; surely she wouldn't need to spend money for medical help. When she mentioned her problem to a neighbor, the woman said, "We have lots of sand fleas here, and the people who lived in that house had a whole bunch of dogs. I think you're allergic to flea bites!"

Allergic she certainly was. She sat down to write to her mother, thinking it would be interesting to count the bites on one leg so as to have something to report. When she reached fifty bites on one leg and hadn't even gotten from her foot to her knee, she gave up. Though the allergy decreased somewhat, she suffered with bites during the entire stay in Mendocino. "I feel like a spotted leopard," she laughed.

Stan had some difficulty with the fleas, but not as much. Astonishingly, red-haired Jacquee seemed immune. Stan and Helen would lie in their bed, listening to the mournful foghorns on the bay and, in the light shining through the windows, watching the fleas jumping from one place to another on the ceiling and walls. Adding to their misery was the fact that they had never yet been able to buy sufficient bedding. The chill dampness penetrated their bedclothes. Worried about Jacquee, they piled their coats on top of her little blankets.

Another complication in the Mendocino house was that the incessant dampness wreaked havoc on Helen's only black "meeting" dress, the one she had to wear to every night meeting and often on Sabbaths. It would be years before unshrinkable, unwrinkling polyester would be invented. Her dress was the standard, inexpensive black crepe that related very poorly to the climate. After it had hung in the closet for the first days of settling and Helen had attempted to don it for a meeting, she was horrified.

"Stan!" she called. "What in the world is the matter with this dress? I don't think I've gained any weight."

He surveyed the situation, unable to keep a twinkle from his eye and the beginnings of a grin on his lips. There she stood, his tall Helen, queenly and graceful, with a dress bulging at the seams and ending somewhere above her knees.

"Well—it must have shrunk from the dampness," he told her.

"What will I *do?*" she wailed. Then, answering her own question, she declared, "I'll press it and press it and see what happens."

Suiting the action to the word, she got the ironing board out. Fortunately, pressing did loosen the seams and lengthen the skirt—but black crepe always took poorly to much pressing. It became shiny and slick-looking. As the weeks passed and Helen had to press the dress for every wearing, she was afraid people could see themselves reflected in the material.

After part of a Japanese submarine and the remains of a Japanese soldier washed up on the nearby beach, all the citizens took turns keeping a twenty-four-hour vigil. Busy though he was with meetings, Stan took one all-night shift a week in the lighthouse. Helen, along with all other American housewives, learned to contrive blackout curtains so that at night no windows showed the least crack of light. An air of fear and uncertainty prevailed throughout the United States. People came to the meetings in search of reassurance and security. Stan could have given Bible studies twenty-four hours a day. They got used to being chronically exhausted.

But when they held their closing baptism, it all seemed so glorious, so worthwhile, that they forgot the hard parts. Helen, however, had a rude awakening when she found that she had all the wet baptismal robes to care for, in addition to moving on to their next location—Willits. In the damp fog, nothing ever really dried thoroughly.

One bright spot that she always associated with Willits was her first large cooking kettle with matching lid. She and Stan had started their married life with a few old cooking pans that Harry and Eula had given them; they were very grateful to have them. But when Helen needed to cook for more than two people, she had to use several pans for the same vegetable, since the pans were small. It wasn't easy. Now she could cook a large kettle of potatoes at one time. The senior evangelist, Elder Warren Wittenberg, had just lost his wife in death. He often ate with the young Jeffersons. He was kind; he noticed Helen's pitiful cooking situation and presented her with another big kettle. Now she was really "in business."

"Stan, I just love this house!" Helen exclaimed, her blue eyes dancing, when they drove up to the little home they would have in Willits. It already had some pretty drapes in some of the rooms. "I can put orange crates on the back porch for Jacquee's toys and make gingham curtains for them and . . ."

He smiled fondly. "For your sake, I hope they let us stay here a long time," he told Helen, putting his arms around her and nuzzling her soft cheek.

They were both so happy. They felt so fortunate. They had each other. They had Jacquee. Stan was getting along well in the ministry. They had all of life to look forward to. Helen hadn't the slightest question that Stan would be a success. His study habits, his devotion, his deep-down love of people and God, were so real to her. Who else knew him as well as she did? Who else could evaluate his potential so accurately?

Just when they both began thinking of another child they

couldn't say. Chance remarks began to enter their conversations: "It's a shame to bring up a child alone." "If we're ever going to have another baby, we ought to go ahead before Jacquee gets too big." Then they began to talk in earnest. "We're still in such tight straits financially, it doesn't seem too sensible to order another baby," Stan remarked hesitantly, "yet somehow it seems the right thing."

"I just know we're going to stay here in Willits for at least two years," Helen declared. "This is the best place we've ever had to live in. I agree. We should have another baby."

Full of hope and optimism, they put in their order for a little brother or sister. Now they had to figure out how they would pay their medical bills. They really couldn't afford to put any money in the bank, with Jacquee to feed properly. They pondered and pondered.

One day Stan came home full of joy. "Precious Little Mommy, I've got it all solved. I noticed a sign saying that a company is hiring men to cut and peel redwood for piling. I went to see about it immediately. I've made arrangements to work there during my two weeks' vacation. I'll be paid ten dollars a day."

Helen's blue eyes opened wide. "Only ten dollars for all that hard work, Stan?" she faltered.

"Why, just think—ten days at ten dollars a day means that we'll have a hundred dollars—more than we need for the hospital, so we can buy the things the new baby has to have. It's just an answer to prayer," he told her.

But when, after the first day, he dragged himself home and she saw his exhaustion, she was stricken to the heart. "Sweetheart—was it terrible?" she cried.

Quietly he answered, "Oh, not so bad, but my hands aren't used to that kind of work." Then she noticed that his beautiful hands with the long, artistic fingers were swollen and raw. The redwood bark was so rough, so coarse, that even gloves did not help much, he told her.

"I'm going to soak your hands in warm water and then

massage them," she told him. After his shower, when he lay in the bed, too tired to eat, she rubbed and rubbed his hands, fighting back tears. He shouldn't have to work this hard at a second job, just to pay for what should be their natural right—another child. He grew progressively more exhausted, and so when a steady rain began falling on the seventh day, Helen was relieved. The redwood was too slippery to work with in wet weather.

"Darling, how wonderful that you're through with that awful redwood work," she told him, as she hugged him protectively.

"But we have only sixty dollars instead of a hundred," he reminded her, between kisses. "How will we manage?"

"The Lord will provide somehow," she told him.

During this second pregnancy she wasn't as sick as she had been the first time. She was so profoundly grateful for this blessing that other trials didn't seem so great. But she was still nauseated enough to feel irritable all the time. Then Jacquee contracted a severe case of measles, and even after she was well, she whined for Helen to carry her, particularly on the short trips to the grocery store.

"Jacquee, how many times have I told you to stop that whining!" Helen cried one day when the child had been particularly intransigent. At the hard tone in her voice, the little girl began to sob convulsively. Helen scooped her up, burying her face in the fragrant, curly red hair.

"Mommy's sorry," she whispered. "Mommy doesn't mean to be cross." And she really didn't mean to. It was just that she was always so tired. And there was always so much hard work to be done.

It was, of course, too good to last—the pretty little house, the feeling of semipermanence, the rapport established with the church members. A letter came from the conference office; it had been decided that Stan should go to Reno to assist in an effort. Following the effort, he would become pastor of the Fallon, Nevada, church.

In stunned silence the two young people faced each other. Then Stan smiled. "Snooksie, you'll be living near your parents after all this time. Won't that be nice all the way around? They'll get to know Jacquee, and maybe even the new baby. So you see, it's not all downhill!"

Gulping, Helen agreed, giving him a watery smile. Packing up their few dilapidated possessions, she tried to crush down her very natural feelings of rebellion. But when they got settled in Reno, and she saw how much her mother enjoyed Jacquee and how close they became, a new joy entered her heart. The effort in the hall with veteran evangelist Elder D. R. Schierman went well, though Helen was self-conscious as the pianist, her pregnancy very evident by this time. At that period of history, pregnant women stayed indoors as much as possible, hiding their "secret" from the world. They certainly didn't sit at a piano bench, big as life, and play away, night after night. She always sat on the front seat, sliding onto the piano bench as inconspicuously as she could.

When the effort was over, Stan and Helen took a trip to Fallon, about eighty miles east across the desert. They found a humble little house. But it was almost time for the new baby. Helen had put herself in the care of a doctor in Reno. "Precious Little Mommy," Stan said to her, "I think you'd better move in with your parents until the new baby comes. I don't think I would feel right in having you go to a new doctor when we don't know anything about the hospital facilities in Fallon; it's a pretty small town, you know. And just as soon as you and the new baby are ready, I'll come and get you."

Although agreeing with the wisdom of this plan, Helen could hardly bear to see him go.

"Can you be here when I go into labor?" she begged.

"You know it!" was his quick answer, punctuated with a kiss.

The new baby was due on a Sunday. Stan managed to have someone else take the church service in Fallon on the

Sabbath, and spent the entire day with Helen. When he drove up to the house, she rushed out and hugged him as though she would never let him go. "You don't know how much I've missed you," she whispered, blinking back tears.

"Me, too," he whispered back. Then Jacquee swarmed over him, and the tender moment was past.

As he prepared, sometime after sundown, to drive back to Fallon, Helen suddenly felt that she really couldn't spare him. He hadn't been with her when Jacquee was born. If the new baby followed the same pattern as the first and came exactly on time, tomorrow would be the big day. "Don't you think maybe you'd better not go back?" she asked him.

He hesitated, torn between duty and love. "Snooksie, I have to preach tomorrow night," he told her, "and the truth is that I don't have a sermon, and I can't very well get up in front of the people and stammer around. It's only eighty miles, though, and if you go into labor, then I really wouldn't have to preach—everyone would understand—and I'd head right for Reno. So be sure and let me know the minute it starts."

Ministerial wife that she was, she accepted this arrangement. She went to bed and to sleep—and woke at 2:00 A.M. knowing that she must get to the hospital without the slightest delay. She woke her parents. "Call the doctor, Mother, and tell him I'm on the way to the hospital! Daddy, are you ready to drive me?"

As she stumbled out the front door, she heard her mother on the phone. "How *can* he be in San Francisco? My daughter's going to have her baby any minute!"

Putting down the phone, she exclaimed, "What shall we do, Helen? What shall we do?"

Helen was beyond worrying about anything at this point. "Just explain to the nurse at the hospital when you phone her," she suggested, then she and her father were careening through the strangely dark streets of that city that never sleeps.

Having made connections with the hospital, Helen's mother was assured that a doctor was on duty in the building. Now to alert Stan, who didn't answer his phone. Well, she would call the other worker who was associated with Stan in the effort. Yes, was his reply, he would dress and go to Stan's place and wake him; but he almost failed, for Stan was so deep in exhausted slumber that only massive pounding on his door awoke him. Once aware of what was happening, though, he threw on his clothes and was in his car in a flash, heading toward Reno.

This time he made it. He arrived just before little red-haired Margie was born.

Back in her room, Helen asked him timidly, "Daddy, are you sorry it's another girl? Didn't you want a boy?"

"Little Mommy," he replied tenderly, "what in the world would we have done with a boy? Since I am in the ministry, you have to be alone so much, and I knew it would be much easier for you to have two little girls. So I arranged it this way!"

Helen swallowed the lump in her throat. Dear, dear Stan. He was constitutionally unable to hurt another human being. No matter how much he might have wanted a son, he would never make her feel that she had failed him.

It was October 25, and the hospital was very, very cold. When Helen got back to her room, her teeth were chattering. "Oh, she's going into shock!" one of the nurses exclaimed.

"No, I'm not," Helen declared. "I have on just this little hospital gown and there's not even a blanket on my bed—and you're all bundled up in sweaters." They flew down the halls for blankets.

This time, Stan was just as faithful with his letter writing as he'd been when Jacquee was born. Helen hadn't quite expected that he would be so attentive the second time; after all, they were "old married people" by now. But she was just as much in love with him as on their wedding day; he felt the same. He said, in a letter on October 28, 1942:

> Dearest,
>
> I must be in love with you—that's the only way I can figure it all out. I can see no other reason why I should miss you so!

Then he injected a practical note.

> Our check came today ($201), and I am enclosing a money order for the $65 we owe the hospital.
>
> Remember, dear, I do love you, and you are the most precious thing to me in all the world. Take good care of yourself for me.
>
> Forever your own sweetheart,
> Stan

Since the houses they had been renting were partly furnished (with bare necessities), Stan and Helen hadn't had to face the problem of acquiring much furniture of their own. But now they began to realize that their luck in finding furnished places would not hold out forever. Besides, they deeply longed for some things that were their own. They had put aside each penny and nickel they did not have to use for absolute necessities. Over their mustard greens, they sometimes smiled, "Here's another twenty-five cents for the furniture fund!"

While Helen was recuperating from Margie's birth, Stan and his mother, who was visiting, as a surprise went shopping for a couch, chair, and end table as the basis for their living room. This was a small beginning, but as the years went by they acquired furniture—some beautiful and lovely, in keeping with Helen's artistic tastes, and some, as she phrased it, "Early Disaster Period." Helen's taste was excellent; had it been possible for her to "do" an entire house with expense as no obstacle, she would have selected French Provincial styles, light and graceful.

Before Stan came from Fallon to get her and the red-haired babies, Helen's mother said to her, "Helen, I want you to have my piano. You and Stan are so heavily involved with music; I know it will be such a help to you in your work, and, well, I just want you to have it."

But Helen couldn't bring herself to take it. Thinking of the long years of her mother's illnesses and that she had never really been well enough to leave the house too often, she felt that it would be selfish to take the one joy in her mother's life. The latter had taught herself to play simple hymns. Nearly every day she sat at the piano, playing and singing softly.

"Mother dear, I want to visualize you sitting here and enjoying your music," Helen told her. "But I will never forget the love that prompted the offer."

Later, Helen would wonder whether she had done the right thing in refusing the piano. Stan was asked to sing constantly. She was his accompanist. She needed to practice. She thought of the songs he sang, the ones that were his favorites: "It Took a Miracle," "The Lord's Prayer," "The Holy City," "The Larger Prayer," and, in the secular field, "Always," "Trees," "Wagon Wheels," and the ones he had sung at their wedding. She loved his voice. She loved to accompany him. But she never felt quite adequate.

In Fallon Stan had such severe sinus headaches that he could hardly keep going. But he refused to slow up, to be easy on himself. The conference president, concerned, suggested that he see a specialist in Reno. After the latter examined Stan, he declared, "I've never seen a worse nose, even on a prizefighter." As a result of the automobile accident several years before, Stan's passages were almost completely blocked. Spurs an inch long had grown back and forth. He had absolutely no drainage. One bone spur had actually grown up into the brain cavity.

"You must have surgery as soon as possible," the specialist told him. It was arranged for the following Thursday. As soon as Stan recovered from the anesthetic, he felt a sense of overpowering freedom and relief.

"You simply can't imagine what we drained from this man's nose," the doctor told him and the anxious Helen, waiting by his bed. And the nose continued to drain.

Stan had been told he could return home on Friday if all

went well. Helen drove him the distance from Reno to Fallon, expecting that he would go to bed at home for several days. But the church was having a "work bee" to clean up the property on Sunday. It was unthinkable to the members and Stan that he not work as hard as or harder than they; after all, he had to prove his calling to this ministry, didn't he?

"Stan, you just can't go!" Helen wept, to no avail. Her tears made him gruff, as they always did. She wondered why she couldn't learn not to weep; she could make her point so much more effectively, she thought, if she could learn to be calm. But how could she be calm when she was so worried about him?

Stan drove the tractor all day in the icy wind and snow that only the high desert winter can provide. When he returned home after dark, he was so weak and exhausted that Helen had to help him into bed. At five o'clock Monday morning he called her.

"Snooksie," he choked in a whisper, "I hate to wake you, but I'm having trouble."

He was hemorrhaging—so violently that soon the bathtub was full of blood-soaked towels. Helen frantically tried to phone a doctor, but each one she called said, "Mrs. Jefferson, the highway patrol says the wind has drifted the snow across the roads so badly that it will be hours before they are passable."

Almost beside herself with fear, Helen phoned the male church school teacher who had a nursing background. He fought his way valiantly through the blizzard, bringing surgical gauze, with which he packed Stan's nose. Helen couldn't believe it, as literally yards of gauze disappeared into his nose.

"Now you must keep your head back on these pillows and stay absolutely still," the teacher told him sternly. By now Stan was so weak from loss of blood that he was completely amenable to any suggestions.

Helen, still weak herself from Margie's birth only six

weeks before, and with 2-year-old Jacquee to care for, surveyed every towel she owned—all blood-soaked—with despair. How would she ever get the towels clean and usable again? Grimly she set her teeth and began the soaking process in cold water to remove the worst of the blood. She dragged the old washing machine into the kitchen.

Actually, it wasn't as hard a task as she had thought it might be, because as she realized that Stan was still alive, was with her, and had not bled to death, the bloody towels couldn't sink her as they might have done. The faithful teacher helped. The equally faithful old washing machine churned away. But getting all that laundry dry in the small house in winter was a staggering task.

The church members in Fallon were very kind to the struggling young preacher with his tall blue-eyed wife and two tiny redheaded girls. To pad out their scanty grocery budget, members with flocks of chickens brought a never-ending supply of eggs. Helen became something of an authority on the use of eggs.

"Stan, I've fried, boiled, poached, scrambled, and made omelets. I've made timbales, potato salad, macaroni salad, deviled eggs, and eggnogs. I've made soufflés and macaroni and cheese with eggs. I've collected recipes with eggs. Now if you can think of anything else I can do with them, let me know," she chuckled.

"Precious Little Mommy, I never get tired of eating your egg dishes," he said, and he kissed her.

Then an inspiration struck her. She bought some water glass and put the eggs "down" to be kept fresh. Very pleased with herself, she surveyed her work. She couldn't know that years later the medical world would frown upon eggs as a no-no food because of their high cholesterol content. At that time they were the backbone of the Jefferson cuisine.

The seven months in Fallon flew by. Moving time again. But this time there was a solid basis for looking forward to some permanency. Stan was being called to be the pastor of the church in Salt Lake City!

When the call came, the two of them were almost dazed. Why, this meant that Stan was really, really a successful part of the ministry of the Seventh-day Adventist Church! Their years of apprenticeship were over. They had survived. The Lord had richly rewarded all their sacrifices and hardships.

But that was not all. Stan was told he would be ordained before he took the pastorate. Now he would be totally God's man, set aside for a lifetime of service—for ordination is the most solemn event in a minister's professional life. Stan and Helen were almost overawed at the prospect.

"Somehow I feel like Moses—as though I should take the shoes off my feet," Stan told her. She agreed. Were they worthy of what was about to happen? They had seasons of prayer together, asking the Lord to point out anything in their lives that would make them unworthy of being His representatives. It was a very special time, one they would never experience again in quite the same way.

Ordination day dawned. Helen had been wrestling with a tiny, nagging feeling about the ceremony itself. She longed to be by Stan's side, even if ever so briefly, so that she could feel that her commitment was recognized as was his. But in that era an ordainee's wife was not included. So she sat on the front row, as near to him as she could get. A helpful member took care of Margie, but Jacquee sat with her, restless and talkative. Helen, though, was totally transported by the service. She drank in every word of the sermon. She listened to the charge of ordination. Her surroundings seemed unreal.

Suddenly, though, she returned to reality with a jolt. At the conclusion of the ceremony, Stan was to sing "The Holy City." They had practiced it over and over in the church so that everything would go beautifully. Helen's sheet music lay beside her on the pew. But she had not noticed that Jacquee had preempted the music, had played with it, and completely rearranged the pages. Only when she sat down on the piano bench to play the introduction did she realize that the music was hopelessly mixed up. But she must start the chords. Stan was gazing at her trustfully, then fearfully. So she started to play. If only the accompaniment weren't so complex, she told herself in anguish. If only there weren't so many interludes of piano music. If only—if only. She did her best, but it was far from perfect. When they were out of the church, and well-wishers had gone, hot tears rolled down her cheeks.

"I ruined your ordination," she told Stan. Even though he wouldn't even hear of such a thing, she had the old feeling that she wasn't really a fit wife for a minister.

But she would have a new beginning, as the wife of the pastor of the Salt Lake City church.

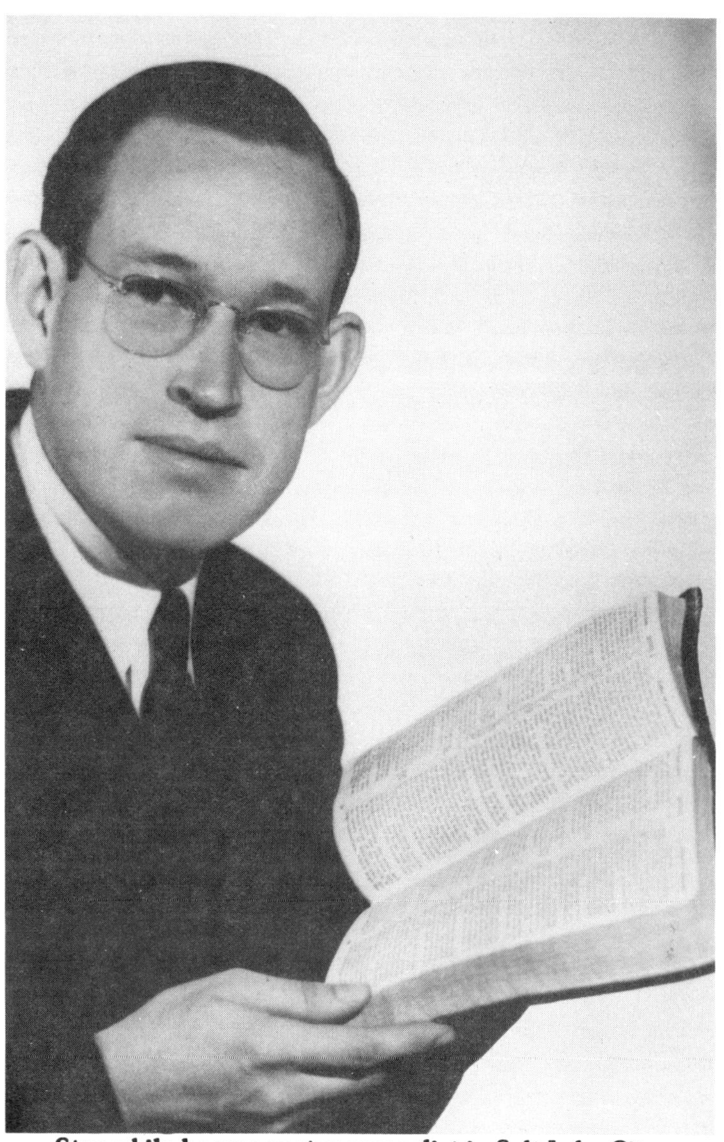

Stan while he was pastor-evangelist in Salt Lake City.

CHAPTER 9
Salt Lake City (Again)

THE new chapter in their lives started out rather inauspiciously for the four Jeffersons. When their meager possessions had been put on the truck for Salt Lake City and they got into their car, Stan remarked tensely, "I hope these tires get us there in one piece." Tires, of course, were unobtainable during the World War II period. He had spent several minutes inspecting a large bulge on the side of one of the rear tires.

"Let's just close our eyes and have a word of prayer, asking God's special help and protection on this trip," he told Helen, which is what they did. God didn't work a miracle for the tire, though, for after about three hundred miles it suddenly blew out and the car lurched violently from side to side. Small Jacquee began screaming in fear. Helen clutched tiny Margie in her arms. Suddenly another thought struck her.

"Oh, Stan, my eggs, my eggs!" she shrieked.

For a moment he wondered whether she had gone into hysteria. Then he burst out laughing, as he safely guided the car to the side of the road. Helen had brought twelve dozen eggs along in the car in water glass—her prize project!

"Is that all you have to worry about?" he teased her.

Helen blushed. They might have been killed, and here she was worrying about her silly eggs! As a matter of fact, not one was broken.

They limped into Salt Lake City at last, on their spare tire, which had almost no rubber on its treads. But they made it.

Helen's high hopes for this new phase of their lives suffered a severe blow when they discovered that housing in

Salt Lake City in wartime was almost unobtainable. They went up one street and down another. They ran down every lead from the tiny motel room in which they were "camping." There was nothing. Nothing had been built in years. Nothing would be built for years to come.

"Daddy, I can't believe the Lord brought us here and brought about your ordination, only to abandon us," Helen choked one night as they huddled together in their bed, whispering lest they wake the baby and little Jacquee.

Stan's strong arms cuddled her close. "Of course He didn't, Snooksie. We'll find something. Just you wait and see."

Helen couldn't do anything else *but* wait—and she felt so ill-equipped for that role. But Stan was right; they did find something. "Something" was about all that could be said for it. Their "mansion" was a tiny apartment on the north side of a building, a one-bedroom duplex. The only place for Jacquee's bed was in a nook behind the refrigerator. (After Jacquee grew up, she would tell her mother she had been so terrified of the black back of the refrigerator that she dreaded bedtime more than anything else.) A table and chairs had to be wedged into one corner of the kitchen. Margie's crib was in their bedroom. Their clothes were stuffed into the two tiny closets the apartment afforded.

Salt Lake City, so beautiful from a distance—and actually so beautiful in the summer—was a different story in winter. Soft coal was the heating fuel at that time, and the soft black soot covered everything. From the beginning, Helen fought a never-ending battle with Stan's white shirts, the only color a self-respecting young minister ever wore. Her sheets became "tattle-tale gray," in that day and age a shocking condition for a housewife worth her salt. There was a dark, cold basement with no laundry trays, just faucets, so that Helen bought large washtubs and dipped the water in and out for the many rinsings, after using the old washing machine, which was still operating. When the clothes seemed dingier than usual, she used bleach. Her hands were raw, actually bleeding some of the time, with so many shirts, diapers, and sheets to wash. (Finding soap was another problem—it was a wartime casualty.)

As if all these problems were not enough for one time, the eczema that had sometimes plagued Helen as a child returned, probably as the result of so much immersion in water and exposure to strong soaps, so much dishwashing and floor scrubbing. Though she controlled the almost unbearable itching and refused to scratch her hands in the daytime, she would often waken with her hands clawed raw, so that flecks of blood were visible.

"I'm going to wear old gloves to bed," she declared to Stan, who, the first time he saw her in her nightgown and gloves, could not suppress his smiles, though he praised her ingenuity. But even the gloves weren't protection against her need, in her sleep, to scratch her raw, weeping hands.

Self-conscious and miserable, she tried to hide her hands, even from herself, dreading to see their roughened, scaly texture. "If I had beautiful hands to begin with, it would be bad enough," she told Stan, "but I've always been ashamed of my big, rawboned hands, and now this!"

He kissed her tenderly. "Snooksie," he assured her, "your hands suit me just perfectly. In fact, everything about you suits me to a T."

Dear Stan.

In addition, Margie was something of a feeding problem and was on soy milk. It required sixteen ounces at a feeding instead of eight ounces—double fluid intake. Her elimination wasn't very reliable. Because of the war shortages, rubber panties were unavailable. This meant crib sheet after crib sheet that had to be washed. Sometimes Helen had the feeling that she was nothing but an animated washing machine, an exhausted robot who cooked, cleaned, washed, washed, washed, and tried somehow, someway, to enter into the joys of her husband's ministry. Her clotheslines were always in use; they were always being cleared of, or filled with, baby garments.

Though the little church, which she remembered so well and where her old friends greeted her so warmly, was very dirty and dingy now, attendance was up because a servicemen's center had been established in Salt Lake City to take care of the needs of the Adventist boys in the nearby Army training camp. The Adventist chaplain and his wife, former missionaries in India, were tireless in entertaining the "boys" in their home on Sabbaths and all other days.

Helen longed to be more help in the church, to pull her load. When she expressed this longing to Stan, he said, "But Snooksie, you're the hardest-working person I know. Look at it this way; if you didn't do the things for me that you do, I couldn't be the pastor here. The Lord knows that."

But somehow that didn't seem quite enough to Helen.

As she sat in the little church on Sabbath, Helen sometimes felt almost disoriented. Had she been a single girl here in Salt Lake City just a few years ago? Was she the same girl who had been so lonely, so lonely? In those moments, as she watched Stan on the platform, cuddled baby Margie, and soothed small Jacquee, she felt as though she were the richest of women, the most blessed. What did a few hours of hard clothes-scrubbing each week really amount to? What difference did it make that the apartment was so small she and Stan almost had to establish traffic signals?

And when the church members who had known her as "Helen, the girl who works in the conference office," proudly introduced her with obvious respect and pride as "our pastor's wife," her dreams had indeed come true.

"Little Mommy," Stan said one day, "do you know what I'm going to do? I'm going to start a radio program!"

Helen's reaction was as enthusiastic as he had known it would be.

"Won't it cost a lot?" she asked fearfully, after having flown across the room to kiss and hug him.

"Actually, one of the local stations has offered me some free time, and the conference is backing me. You know how serious-minded most people are with so many of their loved ones overseas. Most of the radio stations are trying to get more religious and inspirational material into their schedules," he told her.

After much planning the radio program became a reality. Helen played the piano; Stan sang a solo, then he gave a short sermon. Between being nervous lest she strike wrong notes and terrified lest Jacquee disrupt the program, Helen was always limp after the weekly program. While they had been able to "farm out" baby Margie, at first there seemed no one in a position to keep Jacquee for that particular period of time.

The first time they appeared at the radio station with the little red-haired 3½-year-old in tow, the technicians were aghast. "You can't have her in the studio while you're broadcasting!" they remonstrated. "She might cry—run around. Who knows what she might do?"

Stan was firm. "We've explained about the program to our little girl. She knows that when we put our finger across our lips, she must be absolutely still until the program is over." Jacquee came through with flying colors. Not once did she disgrace herself or them. Helen was meticulous about taking her to the bathroom just before the program began, however!

Later, when their college friend Melvin Adams was pastor in Ogden, the two young preachers joined forces and were on five Utah stations. By now they had "graduated" to using King's Heralds quartet music for the "specials."

Being a Seventh-day Adventist minister in Salt Lake City—or in any part of Utah, for that matter—was not for the faint of heart. Utah was the nearest thing to a "church-state" that the United States had, as Helen had learned when she was a single girl in the office there. The beautiful temple and tabernacle with its world-renowned choir and magnificent organ had a powerful appeal. The city was divided into "wards," with a "ward church" in each area; the strong young people's work and emphasis on the family made it almost impossible for members to renounce their connection.

Again Helen was sad, as she had been previously. "If we can just stay here in Salt Lake City for a long time, I think we will get to know the people well enough to make a breakthrough," she told Stan. "The problem is that the work is so hard that preachers leave rapidly, one after another. There's no continuity. The church members are in a mood of defeat."

He agreed with her. Salt Lake City and all Utah was as much a mission field as though it were on another continent.

He and another young minister, Jack Provonsha, bravely fixed up an abandoned store, decorating the front as artistically as possible. They took out newspaper space for advertising, though the Mormon editors were very uneasy about permitting such "heresy" to be advertised in their papers. They had handbills printed, and rounded up the church members to circulate the bills to as many homes as possible in that large city.

Working tirelessly night after night, they prayed even more than they worked. Finally five people were baptized.

"Actually," Stan told Helen, "these five represent about fifty in a different sort of place. I have heard so many terrible stories of family persecution when a Mormon attempts to leave that church that I really applaud the courage of the five." One lady with five boys was so persecuted for years that her life was hardly worth living. But she did not renounce her newfound faith.

During one of the summers a severe epidemic of poliomyelitis swept Salt Lake City. Polio was a hot-weather hazard of the entire United States in those days before the Salk vaccine had been invented. The newspapers cautioned people to keep flies and mosquitoes out of their homes, to keep their food immaculately clean, not to get chilled after swimming, and so on. Helen read all the articles with a knot of fear in her chest. Her little red-haired girls seemed so delicate and vulnerable. Margie was still just a baby.

Then the hot weather struck in full force. The tiny apartment, without cross-ventilation, was an oven. The children could not sleep. Neither could Helen and Stan. Every morning, after tossing and turning on hot, sticky sheets, the four of them faced the new day exhausted, gritty-eyed, almost in despair.

"Snooksie," Stan said one morning when things looked especially bad, "I have an idea! Let's move our bed and Jacquee's bed and Margie's crib down into the basement. I know it's certainly about as unfancy a place as you'll ever see, but it will be relatively cool—or if not cool, at least not as hot as here."

Helen was ready to try anything. She had been spending night after night lying in bed with her arm through the bars of Margie's crib, rubbing, rubbing, rubbing the tiny arms and legs as Margie tossed and turned and whimpered her distress. Later she would wonder if the baby had had a mild case of polio that had gone undetected.

The two of them wrestled the beds down the narrow stairs. For the first time in weeks, they began to have a few hours' uninterrupted rest. Things were looking better. Stan's church ministry didn't seem so taxing. Helen's endless washing wasn't quite so impossible.

The weeks went by. Summer was almost over. One morning when Helen awoke she hurt so from head to foot that she could hardly move. She said nothing to Stan. Perhaps it was a temporary thing and would pass over. But as the day wore on, she became worse. With dawning panic, she remembered a list of polio symptoms she had read in one of the newspapers. One symptom stood out in her mind.

"If you bend your head a certain way, and you can feel the muscles knot clear down to your heels, you have polio."

Fearfully she gathered her courage. She bent her head in the prescribed manner. She felt her muscles knot to her toes. Stan was just coming into the house. She flew to him, as fast as she could with her body in torment.

"Stan, I think I have polio!" she gasped.

He was startled and frightened, but he tried to reassure her. "Now it may not be polio, Snooksie," he soothed. "After all, surely polio isn't the only disease that would make you feel just that way. Don't be scared; I'm here."

What a comfort his presence was! How wonderful his calmness and love!

They had planned to bring all the beds back up the stairs into the bedrooms that evening. "Maybe we ought not to try to do this, since you feel so bad," Stan told her.

"Oh, no, I want to get the house back together, because who knows what the future holds?" Helen urged.

She found that her arms and legs were so weak she could hardly lift. She tried to keep Stan from noticing. She didn't want him to see the tears of pain in her eyes. As they struggled with the unwieldy articles of furniture, suddenly there was a crash. Helen was afraid to look. Sure enough, they had knocked over the tiny narrow cupboard where she kept her only pretty possessions—a set of Haviland salt and pepper shakers that a cousin had sent from France (the shakers were shaped like a little boy and girl) and other china and crystal, including a little gold teacup more than a hundred years old. It all lay on the floor in dozens of pieces. All the things she had moved so lovingly, had cared for with such devotion, were gone.

Sick as she was, it was too much. She began to sob. This time her tears didn't annoy Stan. He was stricken to the heart. Here she was, his gallant Snooksie, so brave, so hardworking, so sick. And now the pretty things she loved were gone—gone forever. He could not bear the sadness on her face, the hyacinth eyes swimming in tears. Her artistic nature craved beauty around her. As he held her in his arms his eyes misted over. Dear, dear Snooksie Girl.

When the beds were in place and made, the broken china and crystal swept up, he said, "Snooksie, I hate to leave you, but I have a little errand that I just must do. I'll be back in no time at all."

Helen, suffering intense pain, lay thankfully on the bed to wait for him. When a short time later, she heard the front door open, then a moment of quiet, she wondered what was going on. Then he appeared at the bedroom door. In his hands he held a beautiful crystal bowl and crystal candlesticks.

"Why, Stan—why, darling—where in the world——" Helen was almost speechless.

"I know we can't afford them, but I want you to have something beautiful to enjoy," he told her. The tenderness in his eyes and voice reached to the core of her being.

Through now-happy tears, she held both him and the crystal in her arms. "No matter what gift I may have in my life, these things will always be the best—they will always be what I love most," she told him, between kisses. And they were. She would keep them for the rest of her life.

Still Helen didn't see a doctor. She refused to believe, now that she had thought it over, that she could possibly have polio. She couldn't have it for one especially important reason. If she had it, that would mean that Stan and the tiny redheads were exposed. That simply could not happen. But when, two days later, she tried to lift 11-month-old Margie out of the playpen, and could not do it, her heart pounded with the knowledge she could no longer deny.

Stan was in the bedroom, putting a sermon together. Helen crept to the door. "Stan, we must get a doctor," she choked. Looking at her, he knew the worst.

But even this posed a problem. The wartime shortage of doctors was still acute. Suddenly Stan remembered that a friendly church member had said, when he had inquired, "Yes, Dr. ——— is a good man, and even though he has so many patients that he hardly sleeps or eats, I know he won't refuse to take care of Helen if she is really sick."

It was hours before Stan could reach him by phone. The doctor listened intently to Helen's symptoms and to the fact that she was running a fever. Then he said firmly, "I think there is no doubt your wife does have polio. Ordinarily I would put her in the hospital immediately. But there is not even one hospital bed to be had in all of Salt Lake City—the polio cases multiply each day."

He paused, then went on. "First, she will have to stay absolutely quiet. Someone will have to come and take care of the children. And now, listen to an important part of the treatment. You must restrict her fluids. She may have only thirty-two ounces of fluid a day, including fruit juice and the juice in fresh fruit. She will object to this; she will be thirsty; but she must follow my instructions."

Stan hung up the phone, his face pale. The conversation with the doctor had brought the horror into focus. It was no longer "maybe." His dear Snooksie was a victim of polio. As soon as he got her to bed, he phoned both mothers. "We have a terrible crisis," he told them. Both instantly offered to come at once. They knew that Stan and Helen, independent and self-reliant, would never ask for help unless they were desperate.

Now Helen entered a world of shadows. She longed for glass after glass of cold, clear water, for icy orange juice, for tart tomato juice. But Stan and the two mothers followed the doctor's instructions.

In almost unendurable pain, night and day, Helen wept in despair. "Whoever heard of a patient not being given all the liquid he wants?" she raged. "It doesn't make any sense; it doesn't make any sense!"

But her family felt that the only slender thread of hope to which they could cling was the doctor's firm assurance that he knew what he was doing. At last the doctor was able to come up to the house and examine her. Even before she opened her mouth to tell him of her violent thirst, he said, "Mrs. Jefferson, no one really knows much about polio. Someday they will, I am sure. But the one thing we do know is that a buildup of fluid in the spinal column causes the paralysis. I have come to the conclusion that if I can keep the fluid balance low until all the germs run their course, paralysis just may not occur."

In spite of herself, Helen could not dispute his reasoning. She had spent hours of terror wondering whether she would spend the rest of her life in a wheelchair as had President Franklin D. Roosevelt. Worse yet, if her lungs became paralyzed, would she be in an iron lung? How would Stan and the little girls manage? For that matter, what if they became ill also with the dread disease? Her mind was in torment as the thoughts tumbled through it over and over.

Stan had moved the cribs into the living room. The two grandmothers shared the living-room hide-a-bed couch. The tiny apartment was in a state of siege. But Stan's meetings must be continued. And the basement was full of fresh fruit that Helen had bought for canning. Would all that be a loss? Would they have no fruit for the long winter months? When Helen first became sick, Anne, the Bible worker, came and lovingly canned some of the fruit. The two mothers finished the canning, stepping on each other in the small kitchen of the tiny apartment.

For six weeks the siege went on, with Helen in severe pain; with Anne, the Bible worker, also a nurse, coming in and out to give her fomentations; with the mothers washing, cooking, and feeding the babies. One day Helen went into rebellion. She demanded piece after piece of fresh fruit, reveling in the tangy juice that trickled down her throat. Her fluid balance became very high and when she was put into the bathtub in the evening her muscles began to spasm and then to tighten.

"I'm becoming paralyzed! I shouldn't have eaten so much fruit. Oh, get the doctor, quick!" she cried.

This time he was able to get there quickly; he gave her an injection that seemed to lessen the paralysis.

Finally six weeks had passed. Helen was weak, emaciated, but she was not paralyzed. None of the other family members had gotten the disease.

"At least I've had the fun of teaching Margie to walk," Helen's mother said, just before she left. "In spite of all the hard work and the cramped quarters, this has been a blessed time. And how thankful we are to our dear Lord that you are not paralyzed," she said as she kissed Helen.

They had tried to keep the news of Helen's condition as quiet as possible, fearing that people, afraid of contagion, would boycott Stan's meetings. They did not feel that he would carry germs when he himself seemed in excellent health.

When the grandmas left, small Jacquee began exhibiting quite a bit of temperament. Baby Margie had gotten far more attention than Jacquee could handle. Sibling rivalry, thought Helen wearily. It's always one thing after another.

"I don't know what I'm going to do with this child!" she burst out one day when Jacquee refused her food, whined for hours, and hung on Helen's skirts as she tried to accomplish the bare essentials. Still weak, she had to make every moment of work count.

Stan took the little girl in his arms. "Mommy, she's had two grandmothers at her beck and call," he said gently. "I expect it will be a while before she gets used to reality."

When Helen's doctor had dismissed her as cured, he said, "Mrs. Jefferson, I suspect that you will be in pain for some time to come. You must work as little as possible, thus giving the affected muscles time to regenerate themselves, or you could still suffer some muscular damage."

Helen believed every word he said. But how could a young mother *not* do physical work, especially when she had no automatic conveniences? For three years she suffered severe pain every day of her life; then gradually things began to improve, but it would be many years before the full effects of the polio attack would be over.

Probably her recovery would not have taken so long had the housing situation been different. During the year after her polio bout, the young Jeffersons moved no less than four times in Salt Lake City. Just as they would get settled in one place, the owner would return from the armed services, gather his family (many had doubled up with relatives for the duration), and demand the house that had been rented to Stan and Helen. Some of the homes Helen hated to leave; some she was glad to leave. One place was almost a dream come true—an absolutely new duplex with two bedrooms, lovely wallpaper, and new kitchen and bathroom.

"Oh, I love this!" Helen cried as she stood in the living room. "I hope we can stay forever. I won't even ask for a mansion in heaven if we can stay here."

But they couldn't. Again the old story—owner returning from the war. Finally they ended up in a tiny motel in the middle of a cold, snowy winter. Now Helen had to wash all their clothes in the bathroom sink and try to dry them in the room, with lines crisscrossed and festooned with clothes just above their heads. They lived in an atmosphere of constant cold and dampness.

Baby Margie began coughing. She could not sleep. Helen was alarmed. "Stan, the baby feels feverish," she told him apprehensively. He felt the tiny forehead.

"Maybe it's just something temporary that will soon clear up," he told Helen, more hopefully than he felt.

But it didn't clear up. In a matter of hours the baby was burning with fever, her breathing labored and harsh.

"Oh, Daddy, we have to have a doctor right away," Helen told Stan when he came into the damp little room after his round of visits. "I'm afraid Margie has pneumonia."

He was as alarmed as she as he looked at the suffering baby. Quickly he phoned the doctor who had pulled Helen through polio, but the reply was not what he had hoped for:

"Mr. Jefferson, I don't see how I can come and examine the baby. But from the symptoms you have described, I feel sure she has pneumonia. I have a limited supply of that new drug sulfanilamide at my disposal and it's very effective. I'll phone the drugstore that carries it and you can pick it up. You must give the baby a teaspoonful every four hours—and she has to take lots of liquids so the drug won't damage her kidneys."

Helen, holding the baby, soothing her, tried to interpret the one-sided conversation. When Stan hung up the phone, she cried, "Isn't he coming?"

"Snooksie Girl," Stan answered, putting his arms around both her and Margie, "there's not a doctor in Salt Lake City who isn't working about twenty-four hours a day. So few of them are left. But he has prescribed a new drug that I've heard about, and I honestly think it will cure the baby. We're lucky to have it."

After the drive across town to the drugstore, Stan returned with the precious bottle. But the baby seemed worse as the hours passed. The two of them knelt by the crib of their suffering little one.

"Oh, please, dear Jesus, please make her well," Helen cried in her anguish.

Slowly the sulfanilamide began attacking the pneumonia; slowly the fever began to subside. As the days passed, Margie could breathe more easily. Finally it was over. Margie was well. But it had been too close for comfort.

Then, in the summer, it was Stan's turn. The four of them had been asked to go to the junior camp at Lake Tahoe, which was in California, but was part of the Nevada-Utah Conference territory. It was a rather long distance, but their stay would give Helen time in Reno with her parents, and Stan would conduct several meetings for the small campers. Helen had really looked forward to this trip. She eagerly anticipated seeing again the area that had been part of her childhood. Following camp, they prepared to return to Salt Lake City.

"I'm going to fix us the best lunch for this trip that I possibly can," she told little Jacquee and baby Margie, kissing each of them in turn.

Stan always loved the lunches she fixed. It was fun to be in the car together, cozy and secure, and to relish egg-salad sandwiches and cupcakes and all the rest.

But when Helen offered the food to Stan, he refused it. Her blue eyes opened wide.

"Don't you feel good, honey?" she inquired.

"Well—I just don't feel a bit hungry," he told her.

Anxiously she gazed at him, but she realized that he was not going to say anything more. Somehow the lunch didn't taste quite as good as she had anticipated it would. And Jacquee and Margie seemed fussier than usual. Was something wrong? She touched Stan's cheek.

"Why, you're burning up with fever!" she cried.

"Yes, I think I've picked up some kind of germ," he agreed, but doggedly kept driving until the four of them were back in their little home. Then he collapsed, his fever shooting so high almost immediately that he became delirious.

Helen did not know where to turn. She phoned her conference president.

"Helen, this could be very, very serious," he replied. "I know there have been some cases of Rocky Mountain Spotted Fever here in Salt Lake City."

He thought for a moment. "I'll tell you what I'm going to do. Since it is nearly impossible to get medical care here, I'm going to phone an Adventist doctor in Provo and ask him to come here as fast as possible to examine Stan."

Thankfully Helen hung up the receiver and continued to sponge Stan's burning body with cool cloths. Dr. Smith covered the approximately fifty miles from Provo in record time. He looked grave when he finished his examination.

"I don't think it's Rocky Mountain Spotted Fever," he told Helen, who sank limply into her chair with relief. "It may be a day or so before we know what it really is, though."

The next day Stan broke out in a severe case of measles. He was still very, very sick and weak. Dr. Smith came to see him again. This time he listened to Stan's heart repeatedly. Helen could feel the knot of panic gathering in her stomach.

"Stan," the doctor said, "this case of the measles has left you with a heart murmur. You're going to have to take it easy for several months."

"But," Stan began, "I just don't see how I can do that——"

"Of course he'll take it easy," Helen interrupted. "I'll see to it that he does."

But it wasn't so simple to take it easy in such inferior housing and with a church to pastor and evangelistic meetings to hold.

Sometimes it seemed to Helen that her children were always sick. This she found particularly distressing, for she almost leaned over backward to be a conscientious mother. From the first she had resolved that she would prepare and serve three good meals a day, even if Stan could not be there for all of them. She kept her little girls immaculately clean; she bore the scrub marks of that on her hands!

Once she burst out to a doctor treating one of the girls, "I just don't understand it! Some women let their children run around in all kinds of weather without wraps. They don't feed them properly and don't give them a balanced diet, and yet their children aren't sick as much as mine. It's not fair!"

The doctor smiled sympathetically. "Mrs. Jefferson," he replied, "the mucous membrances of these little redheads are just as delicate as their fair skins. If you weren't as careful as you are, they wouldn't live."

Helen was comforted. She had never thought of it from that angle.

A project Stan was determined to carry through was the redecorating of the small church, inadequate though it was. He even managed to secure the money (miraculously) for red velvet drapes at the windows and baptistry. What an air they gave the little room! Then he turned his attention to the children's divisions in the basement. The curtains at the windows by now were simply dirty, dingy strings. One of the members had a bright idea.

"Let's buy terry toweling by the yard and make curtains in bright colors. Then we can take them down and wash them and won't have to iron them and they'll always look good."

Helen, in her youth and inexperience, was shocked at the suggestion. Terry toweling, indeed! In later life, she would come to realize that the member had been ahead of her time in practical, innovative thinking.

Their supportive and sympathetic conference president felt that somehow the Jeffersons simply must have a decent place to live, after three and a half years. Calling them to his office, he said, "Stan and Helen, if you can find a modest—a very modest—house to buy, we will advance you the money for a down payment."

Helen was struck dumb for a moment. Then she burst out, "A house of our very own? A house that nobody can make us move out of? A house that I can fix up just the way I want it?"

The conference president smiled at her youthful enthusiasm. He knew the struggles the valiant girl had gone through, trying to take proper care of her husband and tiny girls.

When Stan found a little house on one of the hills overlooking Salt Lake City and discovered that the purchase price was comfortably within range of the figure he had been given, he took Helen to see it. In ten seconds she knew how she felt. "I love it, I love it!" she cried through happy tears, hugging Stan and then Jacquee and Margie.

The conference treasurer took care of all the paper work; in short order, they moved in. They moved into heaven, Helen thought, compared to what they'd been living in.

"I thought my wedding day was the happiest day of my life, but this day runs it a close second," Helen told Stan as she busily put shelf paper in the kitchen cupboards, arranged her few linens in the linen closet, and washed her few dishes after taking them out of the boxes where they were so frequently packed.

The conference president came by in the late afternoon as they were settling. Helen greeted him warmly—he was a good friend, an executive who had a deep concern for his workers—and laughingly said, "I'm telling you, if anyone ever mentions the word *moving* to me again, there's going to be a funeral—his or mine. I'm not sure which!"

The president gulped and said nothing. Helen, whirling from room to room, didn't notice the strange look on his face. She was too happy with her new house, her "permanent" home.

The next day the conference president called Stan to his office to tell him that they had received a call for Stan to become pastor of the church in Riverside, California.

CHAPTER 10
Busy Years

SNOOKSIE GIRL, please don't say anything until I've finished," Stan told Helen apprehensively when he returned from the conference office. "I know that at first you're not going to be happy about my news, but after you think it over, I hope you'll feel differently." And then he went on to tell her about the call to the Riverside pastorate.

"But Stan! We've moved, moved, moved. We've just barely gotten into this house—yesterday!"

Helen stopped for a minute. Then her blue eyes filled with tears. "You know I've had this dream of staying in Salt Lake City for a long time and really being missionaries to the Mormons. All these years when I was a girl here and then these past three and a half years I've seen so little progress. We need to *stay!*"

Stan was troubled also. "The brethren feel that this is such a good opportunity for me," he told her softly. "And it seems that Jacquee and Margie are sick all the time in this climate where it's so cold and snowy in winter. Would the Lord have allowed the call to go through at this point if He weren't leading us? We've always said that we'd go wherever the Lord led."

Helen blew her nose. "You're right. There must be a plan in it somewhere, even if I can't see it." She finished drying her eyes. Then her sunny smile broke out. "When do we move—tomorrow?"

Stan hugged her. "That's my Snooksie. No, I think we're going to stay here about six weeks and then take our departure. So at least you can enjoy the house for that long."

Helen telephoned her mother to tell her the news. The

latter was torn between happiness that Stan's abilities were being recognized and sadness that the little family would be farther away.

Stan had to make a trip to California to attend a workers' meeting before he moved his family. Helen wrote to him as follows:

January 8, 1945

Dearest Darling,

The girls have talked of almost nothing but you, constantly asking, "What is he doing now?" They supposed you were in bed by six o'clock and I am sure they went to sleep unconvinced that you weren't already in bed! Each of them fixed up a letter for you. I know very little of their contents. They even stuck on the stamps. It was with a degree of effort that I kept them from sending off a dozen or so.

I just plugged in the fish.

I have taken out the clinkers and refueled.

I have talked to my mother, father, Harry, and Eula on the phone and have learned that my mother will arrive here via bus at 11:35 A.M. Thursday. Dad bought the ticket and came home and gave it to her.

I stood in a mob at Penney's for over half an hour but didn't get any nylons.

I phoned Wolter's Electric, and they are making the necessary correction, which leaves us with a credit of $1.75.

What do you think of a man who goes to California and leaves his wife a car with a dead mouse in the engine? Thanks to Vern (is that your service-station man's name?) he removed it for me. You see, he spotted it first when he was looking for a leak in the heater. The water was running in on the floor of the car. He put a twenty-five-cent can of stuff in the radiator and it stopped again. I saw it on the way home, so didn't lose enough to hurt anything.

The mouse? It was on the pan under the engine, and I was glad he threw it out for me. Otherwise I am afraid I would be walking until you came home. (Isn't that a terrific sentence?)

I'm not going to start sewing for a while.

We've had several calls about the house. One party that saw it Sunday called back, and they have cash. I guess we don't need to worry about it.

I'll be glad when Mother is here and I don't have to go to bed alone.

We love you dearly. Jacquee almost cried after the train left. She didn't want you to go away. Marjorie cried for you when I put her to bed for her rest.

With all my love,
Snooksie

P.S. I love you!

"Helen," her mother had said on the phone when Helen first broke the news of yet another move, "why don't I come and stay with you for a few weeks before you move to California? I could do some sewing for the little girls, and we could have a good visit."

Helen's spirits lightened and soared. Her mother was such fun to be with, so full of energy and enthusiasm, in spite of her physical infirmities. And the time together proved just as delightful as Helen had known it would be. The pain of packing up and moving again was ameliorated to some degree by her mother's sturdy common sense. Moreover, the two of them bought sixteen little lengths of pretty cotton prints and made eight dresses for Jacquee and eight for Margie.

"You won't have to worry about clothes for the girls for a while," Helen's mother said with satisfaction. "Now that they're getting older, you can enter into the church work more fully. And it really was clever that you chose patterns that button down the front, because this means that when you have to take them to church or other places, you can get them ready all except their dresses, put on their bathrobes, then get yourself ready, and whip their little dresses on at the

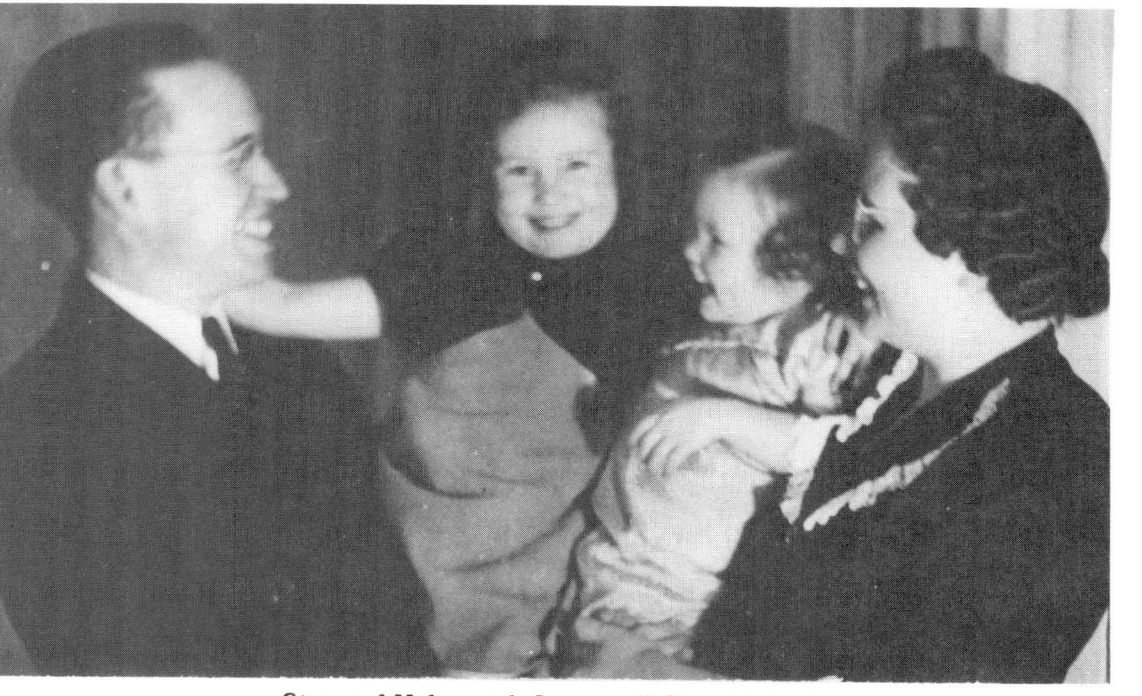

Stan and Helen with Jacquee (left) and Margie.

last minute. They'll look as fresh and unwrinkled as daisies."

Later on, when permanent-pressed material was invented, Helen would think often of those sixteen little dresses and the hours she had spent washing, starching, sprinkling down, and ironing them during that first year in Riverside. But she also thought many times of that first real home in Salt Lake City and sometimes dreamed of how their lives might have been different if they had stayed there.

When they sold the house, for the first time since their marriage they had a tiny sum of money at their disposal. Stan told Helen exactly what they were going to do with a portion of it.

"Snooksie Girl, you haven't had a new thing to wear since we were married," he told her, "and now that's going to be changed. We're going to go to a nice store and buy you a pretty dress and a new coat with a fur collar. Now what do you think of that?"

"Oh, I think it's wonderful!" Helen cried. "But should we spend the money that way? Shouldn't we save it?"

Stan gazed at her lovingly. "No, we shouldn't. I want my wife to look as pretty as she really is when we go to Riverside."

The two of them reveled in the unaccustomed luxury of shopping in a nice department store, of spending time comparing this dress with that dress, this coat with that coat. When she saw Stan's obvious delight in both the dress and coat, Helen's heart was so full of love for him she could hardly contain it. Dear, generous Stan. Was there another woman on earth so lucky as she?

While they lived in Yuba City, Stan had performed a near-miracle, automotively speaking. He'd gotten acquainted with the "right" people and negotiated carefully and intelligently and succeeded in selling the old "clunker" for a bit more than they'd paid for it in Mount Shasta. First, though, he'd found a sympathetic car dealer who wanted to do something nice for a struggling young preacher. The "something nice" was a new Chevrolet sedan at cost, which Stan, through all sorts of arranging, managed to have driven out to him, from the Detroit factory, by two students. Now it seemed time to have another car; Stan literally lived in his car, with all his visiting and meetings. His new post of duty would mean even more driving. But with the war still barely over, cars were still the most scarce of commodities.

While he was turning this problem over in his mind, in the paper one day he saw a large advertisement from a dealer who glowingly promised to take orders for "almost immediate" delivery of new cars. Stan literally threw himself into his car and rushed to the dealer.

The latter's eyes brightened when he saw the well-kept Chevrolet sedan. Upon learning of Stan's occupation, he drawled, "Why, I'd like to do something for a young preacher. I tell you what—you give me your car in trade right now, and I'll have a new car for you in nothing flat."

Delighted, Stan came home to tell Helen about their good fortune. She listened carefully. Then her always acute business sense came to the fore. "Honey," she told him, "I think it should be written into the contract that since they're taking our car in trade, they will provide us a car until the new one arrives."

Stan glanced at her, surprised. "But the dealer said he'd have the car for us in just a few days. It's in a freight car here in Salt Lake City. We won't be doing any waiting."

Still, Stan acted on Helen's suggestion, and was very glad he did, for a strike intervened and the cars could not be delivered. But the wrecks the dealer provided during the six weeks they were waiting to leave for Riverside were so abominable that they realized they could never start out across the desert that way with their two little girls.

Very well. They would take the train. What they would do when they arrived in Riverside they didn't know.

"I hope we don't all suffocate when we arrive in sunny California," Stan told Helen happily, as the four of them basked in the warmth of the train and the unaccustomed leisure.

"Well, we couldn't leave cold Salt Lake City in light clothes," Helen responded. "As soon as we get there and get at least settled for the night, we can change."

They needn't have worried about warm clothes. They arrived in Riverside during one of the heavy, damp, penetrating fogs that marked this area during some parts of the winter. At once they felt chilled to the marrow of their bones. Moreover, the smudge pots that were lighted each night to keep the groves warm enough so the oranges wouldn't freeze filled the air with an oily, black, thick film, not unlike the soft coal soot of Salt Lake City. Knowing the little girls' predisposition to respiratory infections, and Stan's bronchial difficulties, so prominent since his bout with measles, Helen wondered what she would face next. And they still had to have wheels under them if Stan was to do his work.

His parents, now situated in Baldwin Park, where Elder Jefferson was pastor, lent them a car of very uncertain trustworthiness. But when they themselves had to ask for its return, because of complicated transportation problems, one of the church members, a mechanic, loaned Stan an old Rickenbacker that was so noisy it could be heard almost two blocks away.

Every time she moved from one city to another, Helen with her undying optimism was sure that *this* time she would find delightful housing. The cramped, dirty quarters of yesteryear would be gone forever. The family would be housed in large, airy, clean, fragrant rooms. Well, perhaps they would sometime in the future, but not now.

When they presented themselves at the conference office, the new president said, frowning apologetically, "I guess you people know about wartime housing shortages. The only place we can find to put you at the moment is in a little house out in the country. I hope it won't be too bad."

The country! That didn't sound bad at all. It sounded good. But when the president drove them to the house in his car on a tour of inspection, and Helen saw the sagging building, the dirty rooms, the filthy toilet, and the windows that looked as though they had never been washed during their existence, she felt the old familiar sagging of her spirits. But she didn't say anything. Certainly no wife fit for a minister would complain to the conference president about housing. That would be a "hindrance" to her husband forever!

Stan knew how she felt, though. "Precious Little Mommy," he said tenderly, when the little redheads were finally asleep that night in the motel room, "one of these days we're going to have a nice, clean home, and you won't have to work so hard. That's a promise."

Immediately Helen was contrite. "Honey, forgive me. I know that we're in the Lord's work and there are many more important things than where I live. And I can't expect much during wartime. I don't want to disappoint you, and I don't want to disappoint the Lord."

She went through the now-familiar routine of scrubbing, scrubbing, scrubbing. But the house was so small and so isolated, and transportation remained such a problem, that finally the conference officials decided they must buy a little house for the family. Helen, intensely grateful, still wished that the house hadn't been *quite* so little—less than a thousand square feet. It was situated just across the street from the Southern Pacific Railroad tracks, a line that in those days was intensely active, trains whizzing by at short intervals night and day. The noise was so deafening that if Stan or Helen were talking on the phone when a train went by, he or she simply had to stop talking until it had passed.

The large pepper tree in the back yard provided a bit of shade. Unfortunately, Jacquee was allergic to it, and if she got too near, she suffered severely from hay fever.

One bright spot was that John and Helen Hancock lived just two doors from the Jeffersons, John being the youth director of the Southeastern California Conference. The three Hancock children and the two Jefferson children became firm friends, spending long hours together, seldom getting into the childish squabbles that usually characterize children who spend much time together.

When they had lived in the little "railroad house" for about six months, doing the best they could with the old wrecks of cars they could borrow (the Rickenbacker gave up the ghost rather soon), Stan one day received a letter telling him that the strike was over and he could get his new car in Salt Lake City! When he had read the letter, he shouted, "Snooksie, Snooksie, listen—the car is here! The car is here!"

Helen could not contain herself. "I can't believe it! Oh, are you sure, Stan?" she replied, and upon being assured that he indeed was sure, with one leap she landed on their old dining-room table, a piece of furniture solid as a rock. She proceeded to perform a little impromptu jig, her head bumping against the ceiling.

Jacquee and Margie watched her, their eyes and mouths round as saucers.

"Mommy hasn't gone to pieces," she laughed, as she jumped down and swept them into her arms. "I'm just so happy that after all this time we're going to have a decent car—a nice, shiny, sweet-smelling new car all our very own!"

Jacquee had hated the dilapidated old cars. They'd almost had to force her into them. She and Margie entered into the general rejoicing. They didn't even object when Helen, for once, asked them to stay with Grandma while she and Stan took the bus to Salt Lake City.

Helen never forgot that trip. There were just the two of them. There was the lovely new car. There was a sense of lightness, as though her burdens had been miraculously lifted. The two of them sang as they drove along, they held hands, they wasted a few precious nickels on food in a restaurant instead of sandwiches in the car. Such luxury! It was a little prism of happiness, encapsulated in the time continuum.

Later Helen would think of it as the last completely happy and carefree time she and Stan ever had.

Now she was able to enter much more fully into church work, with the little girls growing up. She could spend time counseling those who needed her. She could teach in the Sabbath school, help in the Dorcas, entertain someone nearly every Sabbath, play the piano for every meeting where a pianist was needed, and do the things that she so loved. The busy years began to roll by.

They had both assumed that somehow, someway, the early financial struggles would disappear and that while they would never have a great deal of money, they would have enough to live simply and comfortably. Yet, frugal as they were, they could hardly stretch Stan's small salary around clothes for four (Stan always had to be well-dressed), and school tuition, and house payments, and car payments, and gasoline, and insurance and medical bills, and—and—and. Stan did quite a lot of singing at weddings and funerals, and sometimes he was paid a few dollars, which always seemed to come at the time they most needed it.

The church was an unusually busy and active one. Many young people from nearby La Sierra College were members. It seemed that activity piled on activity, that Stan was almost never home, for he always was attending board and business meetings, counseling, studying with prospective Adventists, helping with this project and that project. Sometimes Helen thought the two of them never really did talk. They greeted each other in passing.

She did not remember the first time she became conscious that there was a change in Stan.

Gradually, as his Riverside pastoral years progressed, he became more and more nervous. He had severe headaches.

"Honey, can't you stay home tonight and get some extra rest?" Helen implored him more than once when she noticed his weariness and nervousness. He had always in the past been so calm, so stable.

"Mommy, you know I can't," he would tell her, rubbing his eyes tiredly, and massaging the back of his neck. When his headaches and upset stomach persisted for weeks, Helen insisted that he see a doctor. He went willingly, hopeful that he would be given something to make him feel better.

"What did the doctor say?" Helen demanded as soon as he returned.

Stan seemed discouraged and quiet. "Well, he didn't say much. He just said my nerves were acting up and that I ought to get more rest."

"Then that's what you must do," Helen admonished him. This visit to the doctor for "nerves" was the first in a succession of many through the next few years, as Stan's nervousness and tensions increased.

Except for this nagging worry, which Helen pushed to the back of her mind ("He's bound to feel better soon," she told herself), those were the happiest years Stan and Helen knew. He and John Hancock held a large Voice of Youth effort. The Barron brothers assisted, and in later years they told the Jeffersons it was this effort that caused them to determine to enter the ministry themselves.

But by now Stan seemed never to have a day when he felt really well. He was always strained, tightly wound, nervous. And he worried about himself, about his future. This condition brought about a deep wound in Helen. For years she wept over it when she was alone. Stan came home one evening and said to her quietly, "I was anointed this afternoon."

Helen couldn't believe her ears. "What did you say, Stan?" she demanded.

"I was anointed. I just felt that my health is so poor I can't carry on God's work as effectively as I would like to, and so the conference president and a few ministers whom I asked to participate anointed me. I feel that I made the proper preparations—I cleansed my heart of known sin, and I have consecrated myself fully to the Lord."

She was speechless. Then she stammered, "But—but, Stan—I would like to have been there! It seems so strange that I was excluded—"

She could see that he dreaded her probable tears, so she choked them back. But try as she might, she could not understand. Only later would she realize that her Stan, as she knew him, was gradually changing.

"Well, honey, I think you should do what you think is best, and I'll stand by you," she told him sturdily. When he had gone to prayer meeting, she had her own prayer meeting, a long session with the Lord. Had she done something to make Stan more nervous? Was she a drag and not a help to him? Were all the responsibilities of fatherhood, in addition to his ministerial duties, too much for him?

"Dear Lord, please show me how to be a help to Stan. Please show me how to be a soothing influence," she prayed over and over.

When it was arranged that Stan would be the Sabbath school and religious liberty secretary of the Southeastern California Conference, Helen did not realize what an adjustment was in store for her. Always in the past they had been the warm, vital part of a church, in the very center of things. Everything in their lives had revolved around the Sabbath, around its activities and the activities of their very own special church. Now Stan attended a different church each week, and though he urged Helen and the little redheads to accompany him, Helen felt that Jacquee and Margie needed their own regular Sabbath school. She was torn between her love for Stan and her duty to her children.

There was another move—this time to a little house Stan and Helen bought about halfway between Riverside and Arlington. The first time Stan took Helen to look it over, she couldn't contain her enthusiasm. "Oh, I love it, I love it!" she cried, running from room to room, checking on the two bedrooms, den, and *two* fireplaces. "Do you think that we could ever, ever have it? Just look at the big bay window—and the red tile roof!"

Stan smiled indulgently as his tall, blue-eyed "Snooksie" gave full rein to her enthusiasm.

"We still have the money from the little house in Salt Lake City," he reminded her, "and you've saved so carefully. I think that maybe we can just manage it."

At the low price of $9,500, it seemed that all was set; but they hadn't counted on closing costs and escrow fee. When they had bought the house in Salt Lake City, the conference officials had taken care of all that part of the matter.

"I wonder whether anyone our age is as ignorant as we are about things like this," Stan said in chagrin. They had to sit down and figure right to the half-cent, but finally their dream came to pass. They had the house. As Helen looked around her at the sparkling rooms and through the windows at the big field where Jacquee and Margie were already romping, her heart brimmed over with gratitude. She threw her arms around Stan.

"Daddy, I'm so lucky. I have you and the girls and now this lovely, lovely house," she told him. She wasn't at all concerned that their furniture, picked up here and there in secondhand stores, didn't do much for the house.

Not only were the Jeffersons ecstatically happy with the house, but a succession of dogs, cats, kittens, turtles, goldfish—every pet in the spectrum—shared, if not the house, then the yard for the next years. "I don't know why we don't put up a sign out front saying 'Jefferson Zoo,'" Stan remarked one day as he was surrounded by furry creatures on his way into the house.

"Daddy, you know you love the pets as much as we do," Margie scolded him, and he smiled tenderly at this delicate little daughter, so dear to him.

The four of them gardened enthusiastically, producing so many fresh foods that Helen couldn't can and freeze them all, freezing having just come into the picture. In addition, Helen put her artistic talents to full use in landscaping the property and putting in a lawn. When the four of them worked together (when Stan could spend a few hours), Helen thought the property surely should be entitled "The Garden of Eden—Western Annex." A doctor friend built a home nearby with a swimming pool to which the girls were frequently invited. What a beautiful life it was. What a beautiful life it would always be—wouldn't it?

Another strange development began taking place. Stan, always such a superb soloist and quartet member, began flatting so badly that Helen was too embarrassed to accompany him. The first time it happened, she could not believe it. And when, at the end of the meeting, Stan did not refer to it, she broached the subject.

"Stan, did you know you flatted on your solo?" she asked.

He glanced at her in surprise. "You're mistaken," he replied curtly. "It's all your imagination."

Helen felt as though she had received a shower of ice water. Stan never used that tone with her. The next time he was scheduled to sing, she was so nervous that she could hardly put her hands on the keyboard. Again he flatted, this time more decidedly than before. But again he would not admit it or did not seem to realize it. Now when he was asked to sing duets with John Hancock, the two of them having become something of a "duo" in the conference, she was in agony. Her worst fears were realized. And soon the two of them were not asked to sing together.

Next he became confused as to the time in some of his solos, selections that he had sung dozens of times. Strained though their resources were, Helen went out and bought a record of the Lord's Prayer, by Malotte, a solo Stan had sung over and over perfectly for years; she hoped that upon Stan's hearing the time and the pitch, he would improve. But he did not.

She learned that she must not mention his singing to him, for he became first angry, then cold, and did not speak to her for several days unless absolutely necessary. She was bewildered, disoriented. What was happening to Stan?

But in most areas of their lives things went well. Stan was very successful in Sabbath school work. He was one of the first departmental leaders to buy felt in large quantities to make visual devices for children's Sabbath school divisions. He organized classes in "felt-working." He conducted workshops, camps, and other training sessions, and although he was quiet, his trainees were making good use of what they learned. Often he was in Glendale attending departmental meetings put on by the Pacific Union. Also, he began attending departmental meetings in Washington, D.C., at the General Conference once or twice a year. Helen noticed that he listened intently to all the plans and suggestions that were made and came home and put into practice everything he possibly could. He never let up on himself, never took a vacation.

He was away from home a good deal, but was a faithful correspondent. Sometimes it seemed to Helen that now he was able to be more loving in his letters than in person. He seemed so tense in person, like a spring that is wound too tightly. When these thoughts crowded into her mind, she pushed them resolutely aside and went on with her busy, happy life with Jacquee and Margie and her church work.

Then Stan's interests began to gravitate more decidedly toward religious liberty. One day he said to Helen, "Little Mommy, I think I would be completely happy to give the rest of my life to religious liberty. I've always admired Elder W. M. Adams' work in religious liberty so much. It seems to me that this is an area where the church really can be blessed by faithful workers, because if the truth is to be taken to the ends of the earth, we have to have governmental freedom to do so."

Used by now to being a "departmental wife," Helen

happily responded that she agreed, and hoped it would turn out that way if he was sure that's what he wanted. As a matter of fact, she had other worries just about this time that had to be resolved. Physical problems she had struggled with for a number of years caused her doctor in Riverside to inform her that she had no choice but to have a hysterectomy. Stan had worried about her health considerably when he traveled as far away as Washington, D.C. But Helen wasn't happy at the thought of surgery.

"Just think how good you'll feel when it's all over," he told her, and when she came out of the anesthetic and her eyes fastened on a large expanse of pink, she did feel happy, in a disembodied, unreal sort of way. As full consciousness returned, the expanse of pink turned into the most beautiful pink azalea she had ever seen, a gift from Stan. He might not be able to sing as he used to, but he was still loving and thoughtful.

Now Helen made a decision that caused Stan sorrow, yet he agreed that there seemed no other solution. She applied for part-time secretarial work in the conference office. When they first discussed the fact that their mounting school bills and house bills and bills of every sort simply were getting out of hand, he choked, "Little Mommy, I never dreamed that the denomination wouldn't pay us enough so that you couldn't stay home with our babies."

Helen put her arms around him. "While Jacquee and Margie are little, I will work only the hours they are in school, and never summers," she resolved. Even so, there was a subtle shift in their lives. Helen could no longer do the "extras" that had meant so much to family living. She couldn't be as much the firm, warm center of the home as she had formerly been. But the extra money gave her such a sense of freedom from financial worry that she was almost giddy. But her life's dream of working with Stan as a "team" seemed impossible.

When she received her first small paycheck, she brought

it home and threw it in the air, dancing around it. "Now we won't have to worry about making ends meet for this month!" she sang. She still was not interested in luxuries, only in paying the bills and not feeling so pressed and harassed.

As the months wore on, Stan began having trouble making decisions. When Helen would ask him whether the two girls could attend a legitimate school activity, he might harshly retort, "No!" without waiting to hear any of the details. Patiently she would try to explain that the activity was proper in every way. Sometimes she would lose patience, and the two of them would look at each other with hostility. What was happening? And when Stan became so nervous and tossed and turned so violently in his sleep that Helen was wakeful night after night, they decided they must buy twin beds. Helen shed a tear or two. They had always cuddled together in bed, so devotedly and so cozily.

As the two redheads grew, they were in danger, Helen thought, of being spoiled. Everywhere they went, people oohed and aahed. Being PKs (preacher's kids) secured for them more attention than the average child, albeit some of it negative. When Helen thought they had been given too liberal a dose of flattery, she always told them firmly, "Pretty is as pretty does." She had long, earnest talks with them. "More than anything else in this world, I want you to be sweet Christian girls," she told them. She worried lest they feel that their father's calling had circumscribed their lives. She never said to them that they could not do this or that because "Daddy is a preacher." She told Stan, "I don't want to prejudice them against the church because of having their fun spoiled by your work. But more than that, I want them to know the principles on which our conduct is based."

Sometimes Helen thought that the Jeffersons had a bit more than their share of accidents and near-catastrophes. For instance, there was the camp meeting time in Riverside when she accidentally kicked the chrome leg of a table and instantly suffered such pain that she could hardly stand.

"I think I've broken my toe!" she gasped to Stan and the children.

"Shall we take you to the doctor?" he asked anxiously.

"Oh, mercy, no. I have all sorts of things to do. I'll soak it in hot water."

Helen did soak it. She also hobbled around on it for the eight remaining days of the meeting. It became progressively worse. She gave up and consulted their doctor friend.

"I think I broke my toe," she told him, and after he had taken X-rays, he said, "Well, you certainly broke something, but not your toe. You broke a bone in your foot!"

For six weeks during that hot summer, Helen pushed a chair with her knee on it around the hot kitchen. She cooked the meals, canned fruit, washed and ironed—with the outside temperature sometimes 105° F. in the desert climate of Riverside, and nearly as high in the little uninsulated house. Since ironing took at least six hours a week, she was almost incapacitated by the time she finished, in her abnormal-postured condition.

It seemed to Helen that the days were so busy, the weeks so full, that she and Stan seldom talked about anything fundamental for more than a few brief moments at a time. Then they must do something, go somewhere, be ready for something. The girls must study, must be at school, must be at their activities.

When the Jeffersons had lived in Riverside seven years, they began to look for a property within walking distance of La Sierra College. They were not situated near a school (the girls had to be driven to school), and with the equity in the house Helen so loved, perhaps they could find something that would suit their needs. When the girls became academy age, they would go right on to La Sierra Academy. Helen had a few pangs at the thought of leaving her precious house, but Margie and Jacquee were far more important. She might never have another house as nice, but that was not the controlling factor that motivated her.

Just when they were beginning to look in earnest for a house, Stan received a call to become assistant secretary for the religious liberty department of the Pacific Union, which meant that they would have to move to Glendale. The strong inference was made that when Elder Benton, the religious liberty secretary, retired, Stan would take his place.

"Mommy Dearest, what shall we do?" Stan asked her, when the call came.

Helen didn't feel prepared to answer. "I don't know," she said slowly. "We're so happy here in the Riverside area. We're finally getting a few roots down, after all the moving around. The girls are doing so well in school. But if the Lord is calling you, then that's what we must do."

They knelt and prayed together, not once, but many times. "From the time I was a child, I've been fascinated by reading the history of religious persecution and delving into those periods where it was rampant," Stan told her. "I get my deepest satisfaction from working in this part of the Lord's vineyard."

Almost without their making a conscious decision, it was settled. They would go to Glendale. Stan would take the new position. They put their house up for sale. They drove to Glendale, about sixty miles away, and hunted and hunted for housing. Nothing within their price range was available.

"We'll just have to move into an apartment," Helen told Stan and the little girls after a fruitless Sunday of house-hunting. They did. But the months they lived there was a nerve-racking time, especially for Stan. Margie, still a little girl, had always played outside. But now when she took a ball out and threw and bounced it, another apartment-dweller was sure to shout at her. If Stan were home, he found it immensely frustrating to hear his little girl scolded by others, especially since she was a very gentle, well-behaved child. Helen observed his tightening nerves, upset stomach, headaches, and general tenseness. And was it her imagination, or did his face twitch in a strange way? No matter. They had to have a change of living conditions.

"Stan, we must look again for a house," she told him, and he heartily agreed. "Since we have a history of tuberculosis on both sides of the family, I think we ought to try to live up on some of the hillsides surrounding Glendale, if we can find a suitable place there," Helen suggested. When they found, in the little area known as Tujunga, about ten miles from Glendale, a little house they could afford, Helen was ecstatic.

"Maybe you won't have any more of those heavy chest colds that drag you down so badly in winter," she told Stan hopefully.

Drapes were not a part of the purchase price. Helen priced ready-made drapes. After all, they couldn't live in a house with bare windows. Then she priced yardage. She figured out that she could save thirty-five dollars by making the drapes herself. Of course she would have to do this in the evenings when she got home from the part-time secretarial job she had accepted at the Voice of Prophecy. But she was as full of energy and "make do" as ever. Triumphantly she brought the yardage home, did the massive cutting job, and began sewing late one afternoon when she and the girls were at home together. The sewing-machine needle was going so fast it was almost a blur, with Helen feeding the heavy material under the presser foot. Alas, her hand slipped, and the fast-flying needle plunged into her index finger clear to the tip and broke off.

The instant pain was excruciating, to the point where Helen almost went into shock, especially as she viewed the needle in her quivering flesh. Stan was out of town. Helen was shaking but finally drove herself to the emergency room where a doctor removed it.

"Why in the world did this have to happen?" Helen cried. "I hope this doesn't cost much, because if it does it will wipe out all my profit." And that's just what it did. Removal of the needle, plus the aftercare, cost exactly thirty-five dollars.

Helen didn't know whether to laugh or cry. "And that didn't begin to pay for the pain I suffered," she winced, her finger still tender weeks later.

Almost from the first day he entered his religious liberty office in Glendale, Stan was absolutely inundated with work and problems. This was the era of the Green River Ordinance and other similar ordinances, which made it a crime to sell literature from door to door. Adventist colporteurs were in dire straits. The Adventist Church was convinced that the law was unconstitutional. The colporteurs continued to go from door to door with their literature. But this resulted in many arrests and trials, to which religious liberty secretaries were sent to be all the help they could. It was impossible to tell when a call for help might come, both day and night. Stan was on call twenty-four hours a day, seven days a week. When, after several embarrassing occasions on which she had invited dinner guests and Stan had had to leave town precipitously to help a colporteur in trouble, Helen almost gave up entertaining. Family excursions were becoming a thing of the past—that is, excursions that included Stan.

During one year, when their June wedding anniversary was imminent, Stan asked Helen what she would like him to give her for an anniversary gift. It didn't take her an instant to reply.

"I'd like a whole day with you!" she told him.

He crossed the room to hug and kiss her. "Snooksie Girl, I know I've been gone so much that we've hardly had a minute together. And I miss you terribly. You're going to have the present you want. I'm going to take the entire anniversary day off and spend it with you!"

Helen's blue eyes were shining.

"But that's not all," he went on. "You're going to get another present. We're going to go downtown and buy you a brand-new automatic washing machine!"

Now Helen's eyes were so big and round and shining that

Stan had to kiss her again. "A—a new automatic washing machine——"

"Precious Little Mommy, I know how hard it's been all these years for you to keep us looking nice with the old wreck you've been using for so long. You've endured that trial long enough. So we'll have a happy anniversary!"

"Well, I can't say I won't love it, but actually I'll love having you to myself for a day more than anything else," Helen smiled.

Anniversary day came, bright and beautiful and clear. Stan and Helen awoke and exchanged kisses. Helen fixed an especially good breakfast, with hot muffins.

"This is really living!" Stan told her, happily buttering his third muffin. "Will you be ready to go downtown soon?"

Helen assured him that she could go that very minute, if necessary. When they got in the car, Stan suddenly frowned. "Perhaps I ought to go by my office, since I've been out of town for a few days and it was too late last night to check my desk," he told her.

Margie, who was too young for a summer job, was along on the big day. "Daddy," she exclaimed, "I hope you won't stay long in your office."

Stan assured her that he would not. The three of them drove to the office and entered the building, Stan going to his office and Helen and Margie chatting with the switchboard operator. Suddenly they heard hurried steps in the hall. Stan came rushing in, gave Helen a peck on the cheek, and said, "Honey, my secretary will brief you on this crisis. They've made plane reservations for me and are taking me to the airport right now."

So much for the anniversary "together" day.

Helen did get the automatic machine a few days later, but it wasn't quite the same.

Until the Glendale years, Helen had always been delighted with the church schools Jacquee and Margie attended. She was aware of flaws, since this is not a perfect world, but overall, she felt that the girls were receiving the kind of Christian education and grounding in Christian principles she knew to be so important. Now it seemed different. Many of the students in both the church school and the academy seemed to her secular and worldly. Many came from very affluent homes. They were accustomed to special treatment, to having their whims catered to. Discipline was lax, in Helen's view. Jacquee and Margie, used to a structured life, to a strong dedication to God, to family worship, to examining their conduct in the light of God's counsel, were bewildered. Finally Jacquee seemed to make a kind of adjustment and found a few friends with whom she could feel comfortable.

It was not so easy for Margie. Sensitive and shy, she withdrew more and more into herself, afraid of being scorned for her principles and beliefs. As Helen saw the delicate little girl become more sad and lonely, she was cut to the heart. She had not realized how much a parent can suffer when a child is buffeted by the world. Loath as she was to interfere, she asked for a conference with Margie's teacher. It was a reassuring conversation.

"Just be glad Margie is the kind of girl she is," he told her. "If she wanted to be fully accepted, she would have to do things that would negate all the training you have given her. I know it is lonely for her now, but the future is bound to hold something good."

Helen was somewhat comforted. Nonetheless, she would always regret the sad and lonely years Margie spent during that period of her life.

The Jeffersons had never purchased a television set. When the girls were small, Helen had said to them, "Which would you rather do—learn to make music yourselves, or watch other people make it?" She went on to tell them that there was not enough time to do both, and not enough money. The two redheads agreed that they wanted to learn music themselves. They had inherited the strong musical talents of both parents. One of Helen's greatest joys was listening to them practice on the piano that they had at long last been able to afford. As the two girls became more proficient, the house was filled in the late afternoon and early evening with beautiful piano music. Helen loved to listen as she worked in the kitchen or the yard. Her precious redheads. Would life be kind to them?

CHAPTER 11

Foreshadowings

BY THIS time Stan had discontinued singing altogether, he who had done so much singing previously. Sometimes Helen would feel an icy finger touch her heart as she looked at him. What was different about him? What was happening? He seemed to be drifting into a different personality, though it was impossible to put the change into words. He was always sick, though he doggedly continued his work. He seemed not to hear much of what she said, though that could have been merely because he was harassed and tired, she told herself.

On the positive side, he enrolled for a course in constitutional law and did well. Many times a day Helen found herself praying that the Lord would help him to continue to do well in his work. He seemed so vague, so unfocused, so scattered.

His stomach distressed him so much that he could eat almost nothing. He became so thin that Helen could hardly bear to look at him. Yet he was constantly under the care of a doctor. "He isn't being neglected," Helen told herself. She prayed constantly. But she could not mention his condition to Stan too frequently, for he became hostile.

"I don't need criticism, I need your help and understanding!" he shouted at her on one occasion.

Could this be Stan?

People told her that Stan was working too hard. She agreed. But she knew, with a sinking heart, that it was more.

Helen learned to live with uneasiness. Stan's remoteness, his increasing encapsulation in his own thoughts, his constant physical maladies, could have darkened every moment of every day. To have admitted to herself that something was seriously wrong would have brought back the long and agonizing picture of her childhood, her mother's illness, and her fervent prayer before she agreed to marry Stan.

"The Lord won't let this home be ruled by illness as my childhood home was!" she whispered to herself one day as she worked in her kitchen. But the little worm of worry kept wriggling in her mind. "What if God *does* allow it?" was the devil's question, whispered so softly in her ear.

Frightened, she repeated a text that was very dear to her: "'*Though he slay me,* yet will I trust in him.'" The majestic words brought comfort. Her private devotions every day were precious interludes when she felt the love and power of God most vividly. He had not forsaken her, and He never would.

Jacquee and Margie came to her from time to time, puzzled.

"I know Daddy loves us, but sometimes he doesn't seem to hear what we say," they told her. "We feel as though we're just not getting through to him."

Helen responded with a great deal more reassurance than she felt. After all, they were not going to have a sick parent, if she could help it—or at least they were not going to be dominated by sickness.

"Just remember that Daddy has lots on his mind," she told them. "Soul winning is just about the most consuming task in the world, to say nothing of legal problems. He has to meet so many people and keep so many plans and projects in his mind, you can't blame him for not giving the same attention to our little family things," she told them.

"I just wish he wasn't sick all the time," Jacquee remarked wistfully.

Jacquee, with the intensity of her strong, caring, emotional nature, had always idolized her father. She contrived her own pet name for him—"My Daddin' Man." Helen, seeing them together, the tall, brown-eyed father, and the red-haired vivacious girl, would sometimes feel her eyes mist over. She and Stan had been so young when Jacquee was born. They hadn't known even a fraction of what parents ought to know. But Stan had loved his firstborn baby girl wholly; he had held back none of his heart from her.

Sometimes Helen thought that with the four of them it was more Stan and Jacquee, Helen and Margie—but how could that be, since Margie loved him every bit as much as Jacquee did? He had enough love to give to both of them, she told herself. Love is always a miracle.

With Jacquee's wish that Daddy would not be sick Helen could concur wholeheartedly. As for his work, she was entirely sincere in her appraisal of its importance and the secondary role she felt that the family should play. Schooled as she was in the philosophy that the wife of a Seventh-day Adventist minister was the most fortunate person alive, that the financial stringency caused by the cruelly low salaries was something that must be regarded only as a challenge, Helen took her place with complete comfort among the other dedicated wives. After all, she told herself, this life was only transitory. Heaven would be cheap enough at any price. She never wavered from that viewpoint.

The two red-haired girls were a source of endless happiness to Helen. When tiny Margie announced that she was valedictorian of her junior high school graduating class, Helen hugged and kissed her. "Oh, Margie, you've been such a good girl. You've worked and studied so hard. You deserve this honor."

"But Mother," Margie exclaimed, her eyes large and round, "there are so many smart kids in my class. If they had studied hard, there's just no way I would ever have been the valedictorian. Truly!"

Helen laughed and hugged her again. "Be that as it may, Daddy and I would like to give you something extra-special as your graduation gift. What do you think you would like?"

"A dog!" squealed Margie, without hesitation.

And so a tiny miniature dachsund entered the family, just prior to a move into an apartment. Having owned a dog in her childhood, Helen was aware of the problem of housebreaking, but she hadn't anticipated that much of this task would have to take place in an upstairs apartment. Moreover, with such close proximity to neighbors, Prinkette had to be kept on a leash. She was puzzled when she was taken down the stairs and outdoors and admonishings were given—but her leash was not disconnected. Humans were difficult to comprehend.

Early one morning, sensing that she'd better get the canine outdoors rapidly, Helen snapped on her leash, urged her across the floor, went out into the hall, and started down the steps, which were cement, painted to resemble marble. Her shoes were leather, with leather soles. The steps were slick. In a moment, not realizing what had happened, she found herself in a sitting position, with unbearable pain shooting through her hips and legs.

But Prinkette must have the opportunity to attend to her needs. In agony, Helen hobbled outdoors, then dragged herself back upstairs, the tiny dog pulling and jumping on the leash beside her. The girls had gone to school. Stan was out of town. She had to go to work. But that wasn't all. The four of them had been invited to Bishop, a small city about 150 miles away, in the foothills of the mountains, for the Fourth of July weekend. Stan would preach in the Bishop church, and Jacquee and Margie would enjoy the teen-agers of their hosts, Dr. and Mrs. Mason. Everyone had really been looking forward to this break in the routine.

Gulping aspirin, Helen managed to stay at her desk until about three o'clock, when Stan arrived back at the office from his out-of-town trip. She had told herself repeatedly that the pain wouldn't last, that it was just temporary. But "temporary" had stretched out over many hours.

"Daddy," she wept, after she had greeted Stan, "I fell and hurt myself this morning, and I'm in such agony I think I'll have to ask you to take me to the doctor."

Concerned and tender, he helped her to the car. Then there was another hour's wait in the busy doctor's office. After she had been examined, Helen said to the doctor, "I am in terrible pain, but please hurry, because we're driving up to Bishop and we need to get started."

The doctor replied, "You're not going to Bishop. You've not only cracked your tailbone, you've cracked the large sacrum. I'm just glad you don't have paralysis. You're going into the hospital for a while."

"But I can't!" Helen wailed.

Stan took over. "Of course you'll go to the hospital. I'll take you there immediately," he said.

Through her week-long hospitalization, Helen was thankful that she'd insisted Stan and the girls go on to Bishop, for they would have good meals with their hosts, and she didn't have to be concerned on that point. She was concerned, however, that as a part-time employee she wasn't entitled to any sick leave. This would mean a big loss of income just when they needed every cent for the house they were building.

"When can I go back to work?" she pleaded with her doctor.

"Not for two or three weeks," he told her, and she found that even after she returned home she was in such pain that working would have been impossible.

"I am afraid you'll be in pain the rest of your life unless you take proper care of this," her doctor finally said. Nevertheless, Helen went back to work, with the ever-present financial need her spur, suffered intensely, and said nothing. She knew she should have returned to the doctor for surgery, but there was no money—and no time.

But she would feel the effects of the fall for years to come and would finally have to undergo surgery.

While Helen was dedicated completely to Stan's work, she felt that her role should be supportive, not managerial.

Though she realized fully the many facets of his responsibilities, her conviction was that he must cope with his profession. He alone knew what must be done and how. She did not feel qualified to dictate or suggest, as some wives of her acquaintance seemed so free to do. She wanted to cooperate and to lighten his load, but she did not see herself as a full partner. Later on, as the tragedy unfolded, she would sometimes wonder whether she should have taken a more dynamic role, yet knowing that it could not really have changed anything.

Stan's nerves had grown steadily worse. Sometimes he seemed like an open wound, contacts with others and the necessary transactions of living being like salt poured into it. Yet he would not communicate with Helen. He would not discuss his condition or be open about his problems and his feelings. He continued to be loving, thoughtful, and kind—except when Helen displeased him. One thing that annoyed him severely was for Helen to eat candy, which he considered almost a sin. "Don't you have even the slightest self-control?" he would ask her coldly, if he caught her eating even one jellybean.

She wondered whether other people noticed Stan's mannerisms—the quick, jerky movements, the facial twitchings, his inability at times to concentrate when talking to others. It was not a question that she could bring herself to ask anyone else. How could she point out the weaknesses of the person dearest on earth to her? She prayed that somehow others would not notice, that there would be a miracle. She prayed that his work would remain excellent, yet knowing that this was not possible.

Stan's parents had become increasingly concerned.

"I feel absolutely sure that a series of chiropractic treatments would do wonders for you," his father told him again and again. "You say that your neck is so stiff you can hardly turn your head. You need a spinal adjustment."

Stan was totally resistant to these suggestions. "I just

don't have any faith in that sort of thing," he told his father.

Helen's parents, who saw Stan less frequently, were hesitant to comment on the changes that were taking place. At one point Helen's mother asked, diffidently, "Do you think Stan has ever found the right doctor?"

"Mother, he's gone to every doctor in the State of California!" Helen burst out in exaggeration, her fear showing in her voice.

Her mother didn't pursue the topic. "Well, perhaps it's just something temporary that will soon take care of itself," she suggested soothingly.

Stan's fatherhood seemed different than once it had been. His steady, consistent discipline was beginning at times to be inconsistent and irrational. Margie was able to relate to his moods with a fair degree of equanimity; spirited Jacquee, now 16, found it harder. One particularly thorny problem was the fact that he was gone a great deal of the time. Helen, during his absence, had to make all the decisions, including social activities to which the girls were allowed to go. Then when Stan returned, he was very likely to run roughshod over the plans, canceling them all out and leaving the two girls in tears.

"You *cannot* go to that party! I don't care what your mother promised you!" he shouted at Jacquee on one such occasion.

"Mother said I could go and I'm going!" Jacquee shouted back.

In two quick strides he was across the room. He slapped the slight red-haired girl right in the face.

Helen was horrified. Could this be happening in her home? Was this her Stan? Stan could *never* strike his adored Jacquee—but he had. Never in their married life had she interfered in his discipline of the girls, but as she gazed at his face, distorted, his eyes, glazed and unseeing, she stepped in front of Jacquee.

"Stan," she said quietly, "this isn't right. Jacquee is a

good girl, a trustworthy girl. She hasn't asked to do anything unreasonable. I think you should apologize for slapping her."

Mumbling something, he left the room. Helen and Jacquee burst into tears.

"Daddy isn't the same daddy I used to know," Jacquee wept. "Something is the matter. I'm afraid. I'm afraid."

Helen tried to comfort her daughter, but she was sick inside. Couldn't someone somewhere discover what was going wrong with Stan's mind and body? Was there no help in the world for him and for their family?

But in later years Helen would come to believe that the Lord worked miracles for Stan during that time frame. His work was blessed; he was effective. People appeared to have confidence in him. If they noticed his problems, his courtesy and devotion to duty outweighed the negative points.

The understanding continued—that Stan would take over the religious liberty department of the Pacific Union Conference when Elder Benton retired. The latter had unbounded confidence in Stan and considered him almost a son. They traveled together as much as possible, phoning home every night—one or the other. Helen never spoke to Elder Benton of her fears for Stan. Instead, she spent more and more time in prayer.

Then an old physical problem intensified. Stan's stomach went into rebellion. He could eat almost nothing that agreed with him. During the six years that he was assistant religious liberty and temperance director of the Pacific Union, he ate so little that he became painfully thin. The knowledge that he must preach, must appear at court hearings, must plan rallies and conventions, must keep going no matter how he felt, was always with him. He pushed himself to the limit, determined not to surrender to what he considered "nerves."

Elder Benton, at 73, was still very active and very happy. He had no imminent plans for retirement. Stan enjoyed his association with him; Helen was happy when Stan was happy. But she and Stan began to feel that the ten miles from

Glendale Academy was too much for them to cope with.

Actually, Helen would not have minded if they had moved out of the southern California area, where it seemed to her that many Seventh-day Adventists were very lax, very careless, in their attitudes toward church standards. This was a particularly difficult problem for the two girls. Jacquee coped rather well; she was able to be accepted by the group without participating in their more questionable activities. Margie, though, shy and retiring, still found school life difficult. She did not feel accepted. Every Friday night Helen took them to the young people's meeting and sat in the car and waited for them, seething with indignation because parents were not allowed to attend.

"I feel I ought to keep them involved in the church regardless of my own ideas about how things are done," she told Stan, who agreed that her decision was right.

"Stan," Helen said suddenly one night when, miraculously, he was home, "what would you think of our building a house right in Glendale so that the educational problems with the girls would be settled?"

Startled, Stan gazed at her.

"Why, that might work just fine," he replied slowly.

He thought for a moment.

"If we're going to embark on anything so ambitious as that, I think we ought to talk to our union president to be sure that my future is here in Glendale," he suggested.

Helen was taken aback. "Why, when we moved here we were told that that was the plan—that you'd be taking over when Elder Benton retired. Has something changed?"

"I just think we ought to be sure," he insisted.

The two of them asked for an appointment with their union president. As she thought about the coming interview, Helen was uneasily aware that in recent weeks Stan had found himself almost unable to talk on the telephone. Just picking up the phone itself seemed a task beyond him; then he could not get his thoughts together, and there would be long periods of silence when he struggled to put his thoughts into words. In talking face to face with people, he had some of the same difficulty. Did anyone else notice these things? She would soon know, she thought.

The interview seemed reassuring. The union president gave a favorable reaction to Stan's work, and while he pointed out that no elections are ever certain and that committees may have varying ideas, it seemed to Stan and Helen that they could be sufficiently sure of the future so that they could build a house.

"I've had my eye on a couple of small lots on Vallejo Drive," Helen told Stan. "Let's find out whether we could manage the financing of the lots and building of a house when we sell this place."

It worked out. They got the lots. They started to build. They sold their house. They moved into an apartment. Life was beautiful. They were enjoying the idea of their first "custom" home, with all the planning and selecting. They hadn't two extra dimes to rub against each other, but at last they felt they were getting ahead just a bit.

Without warning Elder Benton, who had seemed as strong and indestructible as an old oak tree, had emergency surgery. He didn't survive it. Stan and Helen shed tears for their dear friend and mentor.

During the week after his funeral, the two of them were having lunch in the Glendale Sanitarium cafeteria when one of the officers of the Pacific Union came by their table. He stopped, greeted them, and then said calmly, "Elder Benton's sudden death has left you with a lot of work, Stan. Just hang on for about another month and then you'll be through."

He smiled coolly and moved on through the cafeteria.

Helen could feel her face turning crimson. There was an air of unreality about it all. "Stan," she gasped, "that means you're not going to be the religious liberty secretary! They're going to get someone else!"

Stan's eyes seemed vague and unfocused. He was as remote as though he were alone in the universe. He mumbled something under his breath.

"Don't you understand?" Helen insisted. "We went to the union president. We told him we felt we couldn't continue to live so far from the academy. We explained that Jacquee works here at the hospital and is paying her tuition and saving a little something and that Margie works at the academy in the afternoons after school is over. We told him that since I work here in the union office and our work is here, we wanted to make a move—but *only* if there was some reasonable assurance that we would be staying here."

Still Stan seemed confused, disoriented. Helen took his hand. "Darling," she told him, "you don't have to be the religious liberty secretary for me to love you—you know that. And if that's not the Lord's plan for our lives, then I want to fit in with whatever He wishes and wherever He leads. But if only we weren't half through building the house——!" She broke off, unable to cope with the enormity of the blow. With a leaden heart, she realized that Stan's condition had been noticed by others.

There was nothing to do, however, but to continue with the building, continue to live in the apartment, continue working, and hope against hope that it would still work out, that the union officer who had spoken to them had been mistaken.

But he hadn't been. When the committee met, their decision was that Stan simply was not fitted for the job. Helen knew without the shadow of a doubt that her worst fears were now being realized. Others had seen far more of Stan's deteriorating condition than she had believed. He had entered the work in the union office with such high hopes, such glowing prospects. Now it was all gone. What would they do? Where would they go?

When the final, irrevocable decision had to be accepted —that Stan must leave the work in the Pacific Union—Helen suffered keenly. Stan had so many things going. He had contacted so many people. Relationships had been established. Tentative friendships in high places had been formed. Would his successors carry on with these projects? Would it all be lost? When she expressed these fears to Stan, he wept.

"But there is nothing we can do but pray that the Lord will guide and let nothing be wasted," he told her. They prayed together, as they knelt, that this would be the case.

Stan came home one night with a large bouquet of chrysanthemums for Helen. His self-control deserted him; he threw the flowers on the table and began to sob uncontrollably.

"I've failed my girls; I've failed my girls," he wept over and over. None of their loving reassurances could stop his tears. He went to his and Helen's room and lay on the bed, the bitter tears coursing down his cheeks, hour after hour.

But practical matters must be faced. Stan had been told that he could remain on the payroll of the union until another position could be found for him. Helen was grateful for this. "Now, Stan," she told him, unconsciously squaring her shoulders, "let's get the house finished and move in—it's almost ready, you know—for I can't see cheating Jacquee and Margie of the fun of the only brand-new custom-built house they may ever have. Then when we know where we'll be moving, we'll sell it, and that will be that."

"That will be an awful lot of work for you," Stan demurred. Helen kissed him. "I'm a veteran of the moving business," she smiled, trying to cheer him.

The five months they spent in their pretty little house were the last almost-happy time they would ever have as a family. The view (this was before the large freeway went in) was beautiful, especially at night, when from their hillside they could look out over the twinkling lights.

Sometimes after the girls and Stan had gone to bed, Helen would sit alone in the darkness gazing at the lights. "If you pray hard enough and are brave enough through your trials, somehow the Lord will reverse things and make it all right," she told herself. "I must just get my face set as a flint toward the Lord." Again the text came to her: "Though he slay me, yet will I trust in him."

Suddenly things *were* better—at least on the surface. Stan received a call to become religious liberty and temperance secretary of the Northern California Conference! He would have "one or two other departments also," he told her, but that didn't loom as a greatly significant fact in the general rejoicing.

"We'll be much closer to your parents now," Stan told Helen. "I know how much you miss seeing them often, and they can enjoy the girls."

Even their housing fell into place in the form of a two-story unfinished house in Oakland just half a block from Mills College, which was a lovely area. There was a little lake nearby, big eucalyptus trees, three spacious bedrooms with large bay windows in each one, and a nearby bus stop for Helen, who would be working full time in the conference office.

"I just love this house!" Helen told her little family. "I thought my heart was broken when we sold the new house in Glendale, but here we are with something so pretty and so nice—it just goes to show that the Lord never forsakes us!"

Almost from the first, though, Stan did not seem comfortable in his new job. After the first year, more departments were added to his work. At the end of two years he was carrying six departments. His nerves and body were strained to the limit. He was away from home nearly all the time, desperately trying to keep ahead of the "musts" in his schedule, frantic that he would overlook something of vital importance. The union secretaries, none carrying more than two departments, flailed away constantly at their local conference counterparts, whipping them on to greater and greater endeavors, always mentioning the achievements of the men in the other conferences.

"I just can't manage it all!" Stan cried to Helen more than once.

Troubled, she tried to reassure him. "The Lord doesn't expect you to do more than you can," she told him.

With a flash of humor, he replied, "I'm not worried about the Lord. It's the brethren that have me on the ropes."

Helen told herself that "the brethren" surely could not be aware of his intense pressure. They would not willingly inflict suffering on a worker.

Now a new thread entered the fragile fabric of their lives. Stan, always in the past so idealistic, began to express disillusionment with the church.

"I don't think some of the conference and union leaders really care about some aspects of the work," he told Helen one day.

Shocked at both the statement and his attitude, Helen remonstrated, "Oh, Stan, don't say that! Perhaps you and I just don't see the whole picture."

"Unfortunately, I'm afraid I see enough of it," he replied grimly. "For that matter, one thing I have never felt right about is not being able to make enough money to support my girls. Why can't that be studied by the church?" he demanded.

This was not a new line of thought. Helen had been aware for a long time of Stan's embarrassment and resentment at the fact that she carried a job outside the home.

"Well," she replied slowly, "maybe one of these days things will be different."

He turned away, silent now, his thoughts already elsewhere.

Helen was sick at heart. She did not want to add to his bitterness by telling him how much she had always wanted to work side by side with him, fully assuming the role of pastoral wife, a role that could not be lived to her satisfaction when she had to work outside the home. Stan knew how she felt, however. They had talked of it in the past. It seemed best this time to say nothing more.

It had been decided that Margie would go to Monterey Bay Academy for her junior year, rather than the day academy in Oakland. But how could they let their baby be away from them? Hours of indecision and many tears brought them to the conviction that this was the right place for her. The academy at that time had a strong reputation as a spiritual school, and this was what they wanted for Margie, what she wanted for herself. It was hard, though, for her to leave the pretty room with its pink wallpaper Stan had just finished, working in the middle of the night, sacrificing his sleep.

Then came a heartache so severe that Stan, in his troubled condition, was unable to weather it fully; he was never the same again. Jacquee, brilliant and beautiful, insisted on attending La Sierra College instead of the nearby Pacific Union College, because she had "met someone." He would be attending La Sierra. "I'm not going to be separated from him," she stormed. "We belong together. We're in love."

Reasoning with her did no good. So, against their wishes, Helen and Stan agreed that she might go to La Sierra. When, in October, she announced that she and her "someone" were going to drop out of school and marry, they bitterly reproached themselves.

"If *only* we had sent her to PUC!" Helen wept.

"Are you sure it would have made any difference?" Stan asked.

"But she is just a child, with all her life ahead of her. She isn't mature; he isn't mature; they have no idea of the stresses of marriage. How can we ask the Lord to bless their home when they aren't ready to establish it?" Helen sobbed.

Words were futile, as they so often are when people are very young and very infatuated with each other. In a simple home wedding, Jacquee was married; she and her young husband moved to PUC, and began a precarious, somewhat aimless existence. Margie missed her sister greatly; they had been unusually close. Helen was numb. Stan retreated into his silent world. He did not refer to Jacquee often. His feeling for her was so special that Helen wondered, as time went on, whether he would ever recover from his sadness.

In addition to the constant heartache about Jacquee, Helen realized with a kind of sick terror, that things were going downhill with Stan. By the end of the second year, when so many departments had been added to his load, he told her, "I can't do a good job with any of these departments. There's not time. And there are so many important things to be done."

Helen put her arms around him. He was away from home nearly all the time, never sparing himself. But he was coming to the end of his rope. When one night he started crying uncontrollably and this continued until morning, Helen was terrified. She could not calm him, could not find words to bring solace and comfort.

During these two years he had had endless physical complaints, just as he had had in the past—stomach and neck pains, the facial grimaces, unsteadiness, emotional instability.

After he had been examined by yet another doctor who had been recommended to him as someone who would have "all the answers," Stan came home more troubled than usual. Helen, sensing his mood, didn't want to press him to talk. This could lead only to misunderstanding. Finally, on his own volition, he shared his thoughts.

"The doctor said he thought I might be better off in some other kind of work," he stated softly, tentatively.

Helen was aghast.

"Why, that's the most incredible thing I've ever heard!" she gasped. "You're an ordained minister. You've been consecrated and set aside to do God's work. How does he dare suggest such a thing?"

Stan almost winced at the violence of her reaction.

Hastily he replied, "Well, that's the way I feel too. Maybe, though, we ought to pray about it."

They did, and arose from their knees with the firm conviction that the ministry was his life. At least, Helen thought they shared this conviction. Later on she would wonder whether Stan followed her wishes only because he sensed how desperately important it was to her that he continue with his calling.

Stan had thanked her then, as he had so often done, for her staunch support, faith in him, and encouragement.

But more and more both sets of parents were beginning to voice their concern. Sometimes Helen's nerves would snap when they mentioned it to her.

"I've taken him to so many doctors that I'm sick of trying to find another one!" she told them. "I'll go anywhere, take him to see anybody, do anything that he will do—but he has a mind of his own, don't forget."

Added to his other strains was his feeling of being disliked and discredited in the conference office. When he recounted incidents of what seemed overt cruelty, Helen did not know what to believe. Would Christian workers whose lives were dedicated to spreading the gospel torture a member of their own group who seemed too weak to keep his place in the group? Was he imagining it all? Where did the truth lie? It was all so different, so unlike Stan.

Then he could cope no longer. He wrote a letter of resignation to the conference president, asking that he be given a small district. "I hope," he said in his letter, "that if I move to the country, in the fresh air and a more relaxed setting, my health and nerves will improve."

The conference committee honored his request and appointed him pastor of the Manteca-Escalon district in the San Joaquin Valley, between Fresno and Bakersfield. The two small towns, with their small churches, would be a complete change from the endless travel, programs, and projects that had engaged Stan's time. In spite of difficulties in selling their house (and they finally sold for a lower figure than they should have gotten) and the rigors of packing to move again, and worry as to where she would find employment, with Margie's bills to be paid, Helen felt a lifting of her spirits.

Diffidently Stan asked her one day, "Do you mind terribly that I'm not the success we thought I would be—and not the success that I once was?"

Helen ran and hugged him. "I love you just as you are," she declared. "The two of us together can weather anything. You're going to get well. You just wait and see."

But it wasn't that simple. It wasn't just the two of them. A third, sinister force was moving inexorably between them.

Helen's optimism was sorely tried when the only place they could find in Manteca was a tiny house, totally uninsulated, and so hot in the blazing summer valley that she actually fainted one day when she was ironing. She thought of her parents, who had lived in the same house for fifty-two years. During this time she often retreated into her memories of happier times—the house in Tujunga, when she listed all the Friday-afternoon tasks on slips of paper and put them in a bag for the two girls to select; the house in Glendale when the lawn had needed seeding and Stan had rigged up lights and they'd worked part of the night; the company they had so enjoyed having in all their homes; the large kitchen in the Oakland house that she blocked off into three sections when she scrubbed and waxed it; the closeness of the four of them when, on occasional trips, she'd suggest that the girls ask friends along and they would say, "But it's such fun being with just us." All these memories were precious. Whatever else, they could never be taken away from her.

She began to read more and more in Ellen White's books, so that *The Desire of Ages* became especially precious to her. The description of Christ's sufferings touched her heart. If her Lord was calling upon her to suffer for His sake, why should she complain?

Then they moved again, but Helen was rejoicing; even the packing was a joy, for they had found a lovely little house in the small town. It was cool and insulated. But her back was beginning to give more and more trouble. Now she suffered from sciatica so much of the time that walking was difficult. When she consulted a doctor, he told her he was sure in the future she would have to have surgery as a result of the fall in Glendale.

Stan began to act very strangely now. It was difficult for even Helen to describe what the difference in him was, but he was becoming a different person, less responsive to her affection. He was more and more remote. His facial grimaces were so severe that when all the ministers in Manteca were asked to have their photographs taken, the photographer apologized because he could not get a good full-face shot of Stan and had to settle for a profile view, which surprisingly enough, turned out very well. Stan's arms and legs jerked and twitched constantly. Helen knew, with a sick certainty, that the church members speculated privately as to his condition.

Between the two of them, conflicts now began to erupt. When decisions had to be made, Helen, as she had always done, prayed earnestly, then came to a decision. Stan invariably took the opposite point of view, usually irrationally. Helen felt lonely, isolated. She could not confide in her family—she was too loyal to Stan. Jacquee was married and by now having many tragedies of her own. Margie was in school. Only the Lord was always near, always willing to listen to her heart cry.

Helen thought often of the years in the union office and in the Northern California office. From this point in time, it seemed to her that Stan had suffered severe, punishing blows to his sensitive nature. From her earliest acquaintance with him, one thing had stood out—his unfailing kindness and gentleness to others, and his idealism.

"I don't like to hear people criticized behind their backs," he had once told her. "It seems so unfair, and besides, who knows the real story about anyone? Our Lord never criticized."

Sometimes Helen's mind would drift back to their brief courtship, which hadn't really been a courtship at all. She would remember how she would thrill at the sight of Stan coming toward Graf Hall for meals, always pausing on the porch to comb his hair. She remembered their few parlor dates, the few times they were alone together, the few kisses they had exchanged. It was all so long ago. She would always feel that they should have known each other better when they married—but what was the use in thinking of it all now? He had been loving and affectionate and demonstrative, and she had responded with the warmth of an unusually demonstrative nature. Six feet tall, good physique, dark hair, dark eyes—the boy of her dreams. What had become of him? But no matter what, she knew that she would never feel the same about another human being as she felt about Stan.

Combined with her sorrow at Stan's steady deterioration and her helplessness to understand it, let alone do something about it, was her worry about Jacquee. During the Oakland years, Jacquee had had a little boy, then a year and a half later a baby girl—then a nervous breakdown, and then the collapse of her marriage. Helen felt at times that she was drowning in sorrow. What would become of them all? What new terror did the future hold?

Helen had found a job, finally, in Manteca at the United States Department of Labor. She was involved in the program that controlled the Mexican workers who came in as temporary workers on the farm. Their housing and their feeding were very carefully monitored from her office. And so the days slipped by, Stan doing his best to pastor his churches, Helen coping with her job and her feelings of depression and insecurity.

But Margie was a bright spot. She had completed her academy work with distinction and was through her pre-nursing and now enrolled at Loma Linda University. Petite, loyal Margie, who could always be counted on to do the right thing.

"Stan, the members here in Manteca really love you," Helen said to him one day.

Surprised, he asked, "What makes you think so?"

"Oh, the way they look at you—just everything."

He was hugely pleased. He knew that under his leadership the school had grown and a number of people had been baptized. He was doing his best, limited though he now was. Just when Helen would begin to feel that Stan was better, though, she would notice that he had greater and greater difficulty in finding his texts during his sermons. He would leaf frantically through his Bible as the pause lengthened and the church members squirmed uncomfortably, embarrassed for him.

"It's just that he's been out of this kind of preaching for so long," she would tell herself.

Entertaining the members had now become a problem, for when she would be in the kitchen trying to get the food on the table, Stan would come and stand as close to her as possible, as if for reassurance, leaving the guests by themselves in the living room.

"Stan, go in there and talk to our guests!" she would tell him in an agonized whisper. Sometimes he would go; sometimes he could not seem to make himself do so. Helen tried to cover her embarrassment and act as both host and hostess.

Stan's physical condition worsened. His stomach continued to reject food. He was prone to constant chest congestions. Sometimes, in despair, Helen would fling herself to her knees beside her bed and cry aloud to the Lord, "Oh, can't something help Stan?"

It was not that he did not have constant medical attention. Later she would realize that his symptoms were so scattered, so general, that diagnosis at that point was almost impossible.

One of his doctors had suggested that for his stomach and general allergies he should be put on a very controlled diet for six months. He was given capsules of predigested enzymes a certain number of minutes before each meal. He took more enzymes when he finished eating. At first the only food he was allowed was shredded wheat and raw apple. Gradually one food at a time was added.

When a church picnic was planned during that period, Helen was embarrassed.

"Stan, aren't you going to eat anything but shredded wheat and raw apple?" she asked, wincing.

"I have to stick to this diet and see whether they'll finally figure out what makes me so sick," he replied sadly.

Helen admired his self-control and willpower even while she deplored the necessity of explaining his diet to the church members.

Out of a clear blue sky, Stan received a call to pastor the church in Barstow, about fifty miles from Loma Linda. Later Helen would realize that the call was the work of the president of the Southeastern California Conference, their good friend John Osborn, who was intensely sympathetic to Stan's problems.

"Stan," John told him, "in Barstow you'll be close enough to Loma Linda University so that you can get your M.A. and you'll be able to make an entirely new start."

The prospect was thrilling to Stan. He'd always wanted to do more studying. It never occurred to him that he wouldn't be a minister all the days of his life, no matter how small the churches he might pastor. One took ministerial vows as one took wedding vows—for life.

And so it was with total disbelief that one day Helen heard Stan say, for the first time, "I don't belong in the ministry. I'm not cut out for it. I must change into something else."

Her heart pounding, Helen remonstrated, "But you've always said you loved your work—I don't know how many times you've told me that. You never thought of being anything else, and we're just in the process of moving to Barstow, and you're looking forward to getting your M.A.—"

Stan's eyes seemed to clear at her words. He smiled, shamefacedly.

"You're right, Snooksie. Probably what I need is more education. I'm sure the Lord has a place for me."

Helen quieted her fears. It was natural for him to have self-doubts, she told herself, after all that had happened. But the words lay like stones in her heart.

The move to Barstow quickly proved disastrous. Immediately Stan found problems too difficult for his unsteady condition. There was no church building, only the schoolroom for services. It was way beyond Stan's nervous capacity. In confusion, he went to La Sierra and enrolled in some graduate classes, making the round-trip drive several times a week. Things drifted along, Stan now suddenly almost over the brink, the facial contortions constant, the body jerking, the neck rigid, and his mind far away. But his doctors, whom he consulted regularly, did not suggest brain damage or hopeless illness.

"I must get a job of some kind as soon as possible," Helen had told Stan, once they had settled in the pretty little parsonage. "We have to have money to keep Margie in nursing." Jobs in the small town were hard to come by. Helen, enterprising as ever, drove to San Bernardino and took the examinations for State and Federal office jobs, passing them with flying colors. As she drove to the State offices, her heart was heavy. She remembered the happy years she and Stan and the two little red-haired girls had spent in this very area. Life was so good then, so full of promise. Where had it all gone? What had happened? She felt confused, disoriented.

When, a few days later, she opened the door at the ring of the bell and found a huge State patrolman on her doorstep, she was even more surprised. It turned out that she was being offered the job of secretary to the captain of the highway patrol, who took her grudgingly because she was the only qualified applicant available. He never did resign himself to having a *preacher's* wife in his office and he wasn't at all happy about the restriction he felt Helen's presence placed on their language and general demeanor. However, the young officers treated her with respect and kindness.

One of the other girls in the office solved the mystery of the captain's resentment. "Helen," she said when they were better acquainted, "the captain has always had a kind of 'bar maid' secretary in here before you came. He doesn't know what to make of you!"

The constant moving from one place to another had proved as financially disastrous as it was emotionally trying. Valuing stability and her security as she did, having had so little of these qualities in her childhood, Helen suffered keenly. She was willing to live simply and do without. This was nothing new. But what if the simple living and deprivation did not help—could not counteract the overall effects of what was happening to their lives? As Helen looked around her at their friends who had entered the ministry at the same time she and Stan had entered, and saw the stability that their lives had assumed and the gradually building equity in their homes, she had to fight off feelings of "why us?" Ashamed that such thoughts entered her mind, she could not always free herself of them. Without her prayer life and her constant study of Ellen White's devotional books, she could not, she felt, have gone on.

Life was so different in Barstow. The members were restless. There was little unity. Stan and Helen were liked by some of the members; some only tolerated them. Helen sensed, as she watched Stan, that things were coming to a climax. A cold finger of dread touched her heart.

What was about to happen?

CHAPTER 12
Tragedy

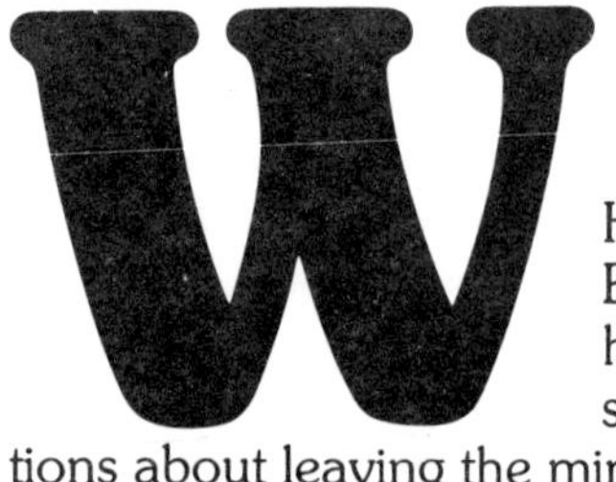

HEN Stan and Helen had been in Barstow only about three months, he began to drop more and more statements into their conversations about leaving the ministry. Helen, who at first had felt she could not endure even the suggestion, could not even entertain the thought, found herself beginning to make adjustments. Well, she said to herself, people can serve God no matter what their work is. Strong laymen are soul winners. If Stan just can't go on with his life, if he can't stand the thought of public ministry and trying to solve other people's problems, then perhaps we are being led in a different direction.

She did not attain this resignation without much prayer, however.

Still she was not aware of what was going on in his mind. The lack of communication that had so troubled her throughout their lives together seemed more pronounced than ever. He said nothing day after day. But he began returning home from his classes in La Sierra later and later.

Helen sat in the living room, night after night, waiting, waiting, her heart in her mouth. Midnight. One o'clock. Two o'clock. When his headlights turned into the driveway, waves of blessed relief washed over her. She envisioned him, broken and bleeding, lying beside the highway, his car a total wreck. Working at the California Highway Patrol office, she was all too familiar with the terrible accidents that were daily occurrences on the highway between Barstow and Riverside.

"Where in the world have you been?" she asked him time after time. "Don't you know that I worry myself to death when you come in so late? I thought something had happened to you—I thought you were dead!"

Her tears left him unmoved, he who had throughout their lives been so tender, so considerate. Sometimes he would mumble a farfetched explanation. Sometimes he would turn away silently, leave the room, and get ready for bed without ever having spoken one word. She would never know then or later where he had spent his time, though as the days raced by, she would come to have suspicions. One resentment she felt were the tickets Stan received for driving 100 miles an hour.

Though at first she had thought he would perhaps forget his determination to leave the ministry, it began to be clear now that some great change in their lives was imminent. One day Helen could stand the strain and pressure no longer. She drove to the conference office in Riverside to talk to the president, Elder Osborn, who was not only a good friend of Stan's but a man of great kindness and understanding.

After only a few words she could not hold back the tears. "Something terrible is happening to Stan," she sobbed in Elder Osborn's office. "He says he is going to leave the ministry; he almost never talks; he doesn't seem to be aware that Margie and I exist; he has lost interest in everything that used to be important to him . . ."

Elder Osborn listened with a heavy heart. Through church members from Barstow he was already aware that things were not as they should be. He had known that it was only a question of time until something had to be done. But he had wanted to give Stan every possible chance.

"I'll come out tomorrow and talk with him," Elder Osborn promised her. He did. He might as well have talked to a stone. Stan was adamant.

"The ministry isn't for me," he declared. "I have failed. That's it."

Nothing John Osborn said made any difference.

After he had driven away from the house, Helen turned

to Stan. As she looked at his face, set as rigidly as though it were carved out of stone, she had a sense of unreality. Could this all be a terrible dream from which she would awaken and find her loving husband, her minister-sweetheart?

Stan's next words shattered any hope of such a miracle.

"I'm leaving," he said unemotionally. "I love you, but I'm leaving."

Uncomprehending, Helen gazed at him. "But you *can't* leave! We're married. We belong together. What will you do? Where will you go?"

"My plans are all made," he told her coolly. "I'm going to take training to drive big moving vans for North American Van Lines."

If the scene until this point had been unreal to Helen, now it was horror. Her Stan, a dedicated minister, becoming a truck driver? Helen had no feelings of arrogance about the ways people made their living; her adored father had been a butcher, a salesman, and had worked at many odd jobs during the depression and after his conversion when Sabbathkeeping was so difficult. But Stan was already ordained; he had held positions of heavy responsibility. The ministry was their *life!*

Exhausted as she was from the many sleepless nights waiting for Stan to come home and from the necessity of keeping up a front before the church members, Helen could not take this blow. She burst into racking sobs.

"What will Jacquee and Margie think? What will become of Margie and me if you leave us? What will the church members think? How much harm will this do to others?"

He turned away, stonily.

Until now, when Margie drove out from Loma Linda, Helen had tried to carry on the illusion that Daddy was simply "sick," as she had done for so many years. Margie accepted this, loving her father deeply, and had waited with her mother for his late return on several occasions. But now the illusion could no longer be maintained.

Things began to fit into place in Helen's mind. She realized that Stan had essentially not been working for the church in recent weeks. He had detached himself from it as completely as possible, while still from time to time appearing on Sabbath. She had had to phone the conference office for guest speakers, fumbling with excuses, her face burning with embarrassment. Now she realized that she must confide in a few of the leading members, must tell them as little as possible, and try to make them see Stan as a sick man.

But is that what people would think? Wouldn't they feel that he was simply forsaking the church and turning his back on all he had believed? Her fears on this point were prophetic; as the weeks and months dragged by, she came to know that this was the general opinion. She and Jacquee and Margie were the only ones who steadfastly insisted that Stan was sick—that there was something terribly wrong. It was a year before their conviction would be proved true.

After Helen's initial shock had receded, during the next few days she tried to reason with Stan. "You don't need to leave our home, Stan," she told him. "I love you more than anything in the world. Jacquee and Margie love you. If you don't want to be a minister, then we can move to—well, say Loma Linda—and you can look for work you think you would like. I can easily get a job there, and Margie is in training there—"

She would hear her words running on and on. Stan made no response, except to reiterate, from time to time, "I'm leaving."

He began sorting out his personal possessions and taking things to the dump, never asking Helen how she felt or whether some of the things would be useful to her. His sense of love and responsibility for her and Margie seemed totally gone.

Now Helen entered a period so dark, so suffocating, that prayer was her only relief and release. Over and over, the words came to her mind, as though they were etched in fire:

"You have failed Stan. This is your fault. If you had been different, this wouldn't have happened. If you hadn't . . . If you had . . ." and the litany went on inside her brain throughout her waking hours. She cried to the Lord for forgiveness if she had failed Stan, and for enough surcease from mental torment to go forward into whatever the future held.

Throughout the next year, until Stan's condition was finally diagnosed, she would carry this sense of crushing personal failure.

One of the bitterest moments of Helen's life came when she knew that she must phone both Stan's parents and hers, alerting them to what was happening, lest they hear rumors from others. The conversations were even worse than she had anticipated, for neither set of parents could comprehend, could internalize the stark, incredible truth—that Stan was leaving, and would listen to no arguments. Worst of all was telling Jacquee, who thought of "My Daddin' Man" as the one dependable element in her own unstable world. "Mother, I'm coming," Jacquee cried into the phone, and she did, confident that she, of all the family, could sway Stan. But she could not. Helen's brother came to assure Stan of his love and support.

Stan's parents drove from their home near Grand Valley to Barstow and spent hours remonstrating with Stan, reasoning with him, begging, pleading. They came away from these bruising sessions in the same despair that Helen faced. "This isn't Stan," his father said over and over. "This isn't Stan."

Stan, who had always been so polite and considerate of his parents, was now brusque, discourteous, uncaring.

Then a tiny glimmer of light penetrated the darkness. During one conversation when Helen urged him to look for work in Loma Linda, Stan—to her complete surprise—suddenly agreed.

"All right," he said, "let's get a paper and see what's

available in the Loma Linda area."

Excitedly Helen secured the paper. She marked several advertisements she thought might suit Stan's capabilities. She phoned for appointments, her heart in her mouth, wondering whether he would go through with the interviews. He did. But each time, when he returned to the car, he announced coldly, "That's not the job for me." Then she began to realize that probably he had consented to the interviews only because of her, because of a lingering sense of responsibility for her wishes.

Sleepless, exhausted, Helen still pushed herself to go to work each day as far as possible. She confided the brief outline of her tragedy to her boss, but felt that since the future seemed so uncertain financially, she must not give up the tiny security her job offered. At least it would put food on the table for Margie and herself and help to pay Margie's school bills.

Stan's facial grimaces, the twitching of his arms and legs, the spasticity in his hands, seemed more pronounced each day. In spite of her natural feelings of resentment at his decision, Helen's heart went out to him. One evening, watching his discomfort as he sat in a chair in the living room, she went and knelt down beside him.

"Daddy dear," she whispered, "won't you let me check you into Loma Linda University Hospital for tests? Surely, surely something can help you."

As he gazed at the blue, blue eyes he had always loved, something of the old Stan came back. He put his arm around Helen and rested his head on her shoulder.

"All right, Little Mommy," he whispered back. "I will do it for you, if you will make all the arrangements."

Helen flew to the phone before he could change his mind. Almost before he knew what was happening, she had a little suitcase packed, had him in the car, and was headed toward Loma Linda. Her heart beating with the first hope in many days, she made the arrangements at the desk, filled out the multitudinous forms, coped with the insurance information, got him settled in his room, alerted Margie, and stayed with her for the night. The two of them knelt together and prayed as they had never prayed before, that the doctors who examined Stan would be given an extra measure of wisdom, of understanding.

"Please, dear Jesus, help the doctors to find out what is wrong with Daddy," Margie prayed, her simple faith bringing fresh tears to Helen's eyes.

For two weeks there were endless tests, endless conferences. Helen shuttled between Barstow and Loma Linda, dazed, exhausted, always in an attitude of prayer, afraid to hope, yet hoping against hope.

Finally Helen was called in for an interview. The physician who spoke to her seemed almost accusatory. "Has your husband changed drastically in the past few weeks?" he demanded.

Confused, Helen tried to answer accurately. What would come under the heading of "drastically"? He had been drifting for so long; his symptoms were only more pronounced than they had been—did the physician mean something terribly dramatic?

"I—I—don't think so," she stammered.

"Then all I can tell you is that he is normal. He is a man who has had a lot of bad luck, he's had professional blows, and he's fed up and made up his mind to leave. That's all I can tell you."

The room whirled around Helen. What was he saying? How could Stan be "normal"?

"No, no, you don't understand!" she cried. But the doctor would hear no more.

"Mrs. Jefferson," he told her firmly, "I have gone over all the tests as carefully as possible. You are welcome to see the results of them. I have other patients waiting. I repeat that I can find nothing abnormal." He turned on his heel and walked out of the room.

Margie, who had been affiliating at the Patton State

Hospital, turned to her mother. "Mommy," she said, "I know—at least I think—that Daddy has Huntington's disease."

That was the first time Helen heard the words "Huntington's disease"—the words that changed her life, that eventually crushed her heart and hopes. But Margie, a student nurse, was not in a position to press her point, and later Helen came to know that of all diseases, Huntington's chorea is one of the most difficult to diagnose, since the symptoms are so scattered and so unspecific and so changing.

When it was time to check Stan out of the hospital, Helen learned that his willingness to be admitted had not been, as she had hoped, regard for her, but his necessity to present a clean bill of health to the truckers' school in Fort Wayne, Indiana. Behind her back, he had made all his arrangements to report there at a specified time, but could be admitted only if his health was pronounced passable. He had let the doctor know that this was his plan and the latter, finding no problems with the tests and thus seeing no reason to refuse, had agreed to fill out the form Stan needed.

Then help from another quarter intervened. A minister friend of Stan's asked for an appointment with the doctor a few days after Stan and Helen were back in Barstow.

"I suppose you think that Mrs. Jefferson is acting as any rejected wife would act," he told the doctor, "but I want you to know that the man you treated is not the Stan Jefferson that all his friends have known. He seems like a total stranger. Can you honestly and safely OK him for a truck drivers' school?"

Obviously this was a new thought to the physician. Obviously he had thought that a marital rift might be the main ingredient in the situation.

"Well," he said slowly, "if you feel as strongly as you do, perhaps we ought to hold up the certificate of health for just a bit."

When Stan phoned the doctor's office and demanded the certificate, the doctor explained his change of mind. Saying nothing more, Stan hung up the phone. He went outside, got in the car, turned out into the driveway with tires screaming, and started for Loma Linda. With no warning, he strode into the doctor's office, past the receptionist, and confronted the doctor.

"You either give me that certificate or I'll kill you," he announced coldly, without a flicker of emotion.

The doctor thought of the safety of his nurses and his other patients. Too late he saw the madness in Stan's eyes, the lack of social responsibility. But it was too late to argue. Silently he handed the certificate to Stan, who just as silently turned and walked out of the office.

With this unexpected evidence of disturbed conduct, the physician contacted Helen. "Perhaps you had better try to commit him to Patton for further tests and evaluations," he told her. Helen fought down the bitterness in her heart. When he was a patient at the hospital, he could have been transferred to Patton with a minimum of arrangements. Now it was all up to her. Besides, did she have the emotional strength to walk into a State mental hospital and commit Stan—her Stan—to whatever might become of him there?

She must try. By this time she was in such a state of shock and horror that she could not take the long drive to San Bernardino by herself. A church member offered to make the trip. By now sympathy and love poured in to Helen from members. Aware of her agony, they tried to ease the pain with flowers, gifts of food, and loving gestures.

Helen thought her heart would beat out of her chest when she walked into the district attorney's office and explained her visit. "I—I—I want to commit my husband," she faltered.

Unemotionally, the district attorney replied, "Committing a patient takes several days."

When Helen did not reply, not knowing what to say, he

asked suspiciously, "Is there a divorce or marital separation involved in this situation?"

Shrinking with humiliation, Helen admitted that a separation was in the making. "In that case," the district attorney told her, "we will not take him. If we took all the husbands or wives whose partner wanted to commit them to an insane asylum when they leave, we'd turn the whole State into one big hospital."

The inference was clear. Helen was taking out her resentment on the husband who was leaving her. Protests would have done no good. She got back in the car, dazed and uncomprehending, and her friend drove her back to the home that was no longer home, to the husband who was no longer her husband.

Stan, unaware of her errand (mercifully, since her safety might have been at stake had he known), announced his plans. He would leave, he said, on July 5, driving to Fort Wayne, where he would enter an upcoming session of training put on by North American Van Lines. (Helen realized now that during many of those nights when she had waited for him, too weary to sit up, too nervous to lie down, too frantic to read, that he had probably been talking to truck drivers at truck stops, getting all the information he could. What else he had been doing, she did not care to speculate on.)

Calmly and coldly he explained his further plans. He would take their new Ford, which was fully paid for—their first car with air conditioning and other comforts. He was also taking the equity they had gotten from their house in Oakland—$6,000, which at that time was a good "nest egg" and which represented a lifetime of sacrifice and saving and doing without on Helen's part. He would have to have this, he told Helen, to purchase a tractor-trailer. She would have an old car, the second mortgage on the house in Oakland, and the furniture in the parsonage where they were living.

"But how will I get Margie through the nurse's course?"

Helen cried. "She is doing so well. All this isn't her fault."

He did not reply. She could not reach him.

Later she would come to believe—and Stan would tell her—that if he had been told that he was indeed sick, he would not have gone. He was in such despair because of the emotions that besieged him, the disorientation, the feeling of failure, the physical manifestations, that in his confused state it seemed to him the only solution was to break with everything he knew.

July 5 was drawing near. The tragic drama was drawing toward its denouement. The last night came. Helen had been given sedative pills by a doctor friend in the church. Members had rallied around her. But on this last night there were just the two of them. At the end of her rope, Helen gulped several of the tranquilizing pills, begging for temporary relief from a pain that was too brutal to be endured. She drifted into merciful sleep.

When she awoke the next morning, Stan was gone. And she knew, with a certainty as though she had been granted a gift of prophecy, that Stan as she knew him—lover, husband, father, dear companion—would never come again.

And now she could not cope, could not go to work, could not carry on the routine of living, could not do what had to be done. From the childhood years with her mother's illness to the young years when she was so alone in Salt Lake City, to the early married years when poverty was a constant companion, through all the years of Stan's illnesses, of his disillusionments, of the embarrassments and disappointments, she had been able to cope. Now she could not. The heart had gone out of her. Even God, her lifelong solace and strength, seemed far away.

Margie enlisted the aid of the church school teacher and his wife, who were holding the church together in addition to their other duties. "I want to take Mother to Glendale and put her in the hospital," Margie told them. "She has to have help to get through this."

For a week Helen existed in a world of half shadows, half reality, blindly swallowing medications that were given her, abandoning her will to that of others in a childlike way. When at the end of the week she began to assume her own personality again, and began the climb back upward from the slough of despondency, she received a bill from a psychiatrist. Startled, she phoned him from her room. "I have no recollection of ever seeing you," she told him. "If you worked with me and helped me, then of course I'll be glad to pay the bill, but otherwise—"

He assured her that they had talked several times and that he felt that he had helped her.

She was told that she could be released from the hospital on Sabbath morning. Before she left, her doctor—the one who had been responsible primarily for her care—came into the room. "Helen," he told her, "my mother was divorced. She thought the end of the world had come. But she was wrong. She married again and is very, very happy. You too can make another life."

But Helen was not yet ready for any such counsel, any such philosophy. She was standing on the brink of a precipice, swaying from side to side emotionally.

Now she had to begin the impossible task of living when there seemed so little to live for. She had to learn to push back the waves of panic that threatened to engulf her. She had to learn to get used to never getting used to the tragedy. She had to learn to live with never being happy.

During the final days Stan and she were together, she had said to him, "Stan, what will I do? Where will I go? How will I make a home for Margie?"

He seemed disinterested, but finally replied, "Well, why don't you just stay here?"

"You know I can't do that!" she exclaimed. "This parsonage belongs to the church. They'll be bringing in a new pastor as soon as possible. He and his family will have to have this place."

He had gazed at her blankly, uncaring—he who had throughout their lifetime been so concerned, so caring, about anything that affected her.

Driving back to Barstow after she had been dismissed from the hospital, Helen's heart seemed bruised by a giant hammer. All too well she realized what a storm of gossip and speculation must now have raced through the conference—through the entire Pacific Union. In the past, when a minister "defected" from his high and holy calling, she realized that she herself had been unduly interested in the details, had not been attuned to the suffering of his wife and family. Now she would have given anything to take back any careless comments she had made.

"If only our friends and acquaintances could realize that Daddy is a very, very sick man," she whispered to Margie. "If only they wouldn't think of him as a person who is being untrue to his vows to the Lord. If only—"

Margie had no answer. Helen knew, with a sick certainty, that others would not believe that he was ill. They would not believe it for many sad years in the future.

She also remembered the days before she had become engaged to Stan, and how earnestly she had prayed that the Lord would direct as to what her answer to his proposal should be. "Lord, the one thing I can't face in a marriage is constant sickness," she had said on her knees. Even standing in the vestibule of the Reno church, listening to the processional for her wedding party, she had prayed one more time: "If there is going to be sickness or unbearable stress in our marriage, please tell me *now*, Lord!"

Could God—would God—have made a mockery of her prayers? All seemed dark; God's throne seemed far away. Panic was about to engulf her. Then into her mind came the words again, rocklike, sure, comforting: "Though he slay me, yet will I trust in him."

Like a swimmer struggling up from the depths, Helen emerged from her despair. The unbelievable had happened.

Life must go on. The new pastor would need the house in August; friends in Glendale at the Pacific Union Conference office contacted Helen with a job offer, which she gratefully accepted. Margie would be affiliating at the White Memorial Hospital in Los Angeles for a year, so it seemed to Helen that it would be best if the two of them situated in Glendale. Already she had said to the petite red-haired girl, "Margie, I don't know how in the world we are going to pay your tuition. We won't get any educational allowance from the conference now that Daddy has dropped out of the ministry, and I guess we won't have anything except the small salary I'll earn and the small checks from the second mortgage on the house in Oakland. But there is one thing I know: God wants you to get your nursing degree."

This goal—Margie's degree—became Helen's motivation for the immediate present. Housing was the first matter to be dealt with. The tiny dachsund (she who had been Helen's "downfall") was still very much a member of the family. Helen and Margie could not think of giving her away and cause themselves a second bereavement. But her presence made many apartments off-limits to them. Providentially they found a tiny house about a block from the Voice of Prophecy building that the two of them, artistic as they were, fixed up. When they moved in, Helen's heart received a new blow as she discovered that a large share of her possessions simply would not fit into the house; they had lived in larger houses for so long she had not realized how small the new house really was. When it was clear to her that not one more object would fit into the four-room house, she said to the movers, "Take the rest of the things with you and keep them yourselves, or give them away." Sadly she and Margie watched as their furniture, bric-a-brac, and objects d'art disappeared back into the moving truck. They never saw those things again.

Their car, which Margie had been using in Loma Linda, was an old 1953 Mercury, in precarious condition. Helen had absolutely no cash for another car and had established no credit of her own; also, this was a time when women were often not allowed to do credit buying themselves. The philosophy prevailed that only males were qualified to handle money. How would Margie get to the White Memorial Hospital, miles across Los Angeles, each day?

The Lord solved the problem almost before they could be concerned about it. "Mother," Margie exclaimed, racing into the little house one day, "two of my classmates live just a few blocks from here. They have a car and I can ride with them!"

Helen breathed a prayer of thankfulness.

Another source of thankfulness was the supportive attitude of John Osborn. His manner made it perfectly clear that Helen could call on him at any time, at any place, and he would do everything in his power to help her. His compassion for her tragedy was boundless. During the final days before Stan's departure, he had tried to work with Helen to get him into Patton, himself convinced that Stan was suffering from an undiagnosed nervous disease. He had helped Helen financially in every way he could legitimately do so.

"If you couldn't see fit to prevent Stan's illness, Lord, then I thank You from the bottom of my heart that Elder Osborn called us to the Southeastern California Conference so that he was here to help me," Helen prayed many times.

Another prayer that was never far from Helen's lips was, "Lord, please, never let any bitterness come into my heart. Please, Lord, keep my heart soft and loving. You died to help me to trust. Please work this miracle in my life."

Now life settled down into a kind of half existence. Helen felt as though she were holding her breath. The days came and went. Margie, clever with her hands, kept Helen's hair beautiful; grief thinned her already good figure down to beautiful proportions. She was resolved not to vegetate and accepted an invitation to be pianist for an effort nearby being held by Dr. Clifford Anderson. At the office she tried to hold her head high, tried to act as though she were unaware of little groups talking together, groups who became suddenly silent when she joined them.

Two other friends were intensely supportive at this time. Mrs. Jack Blacker, whom she and Stan had known in northern California, invited Helen to accompany her on shopping trips. Etta Blacker encouraged her to enroll in a class in millinery, and the two of them smiled together over their attempts at creativity.

Helen was determined to smile, if only on the surface; she knew all too well that long-continued problems and heartaches of others become boring. Besides, she said to herself, people will feel guilty around me when they're smiling and laughing if I'm always long-faced.

But that didn't take care of the sleepless nights. She would toss and turn, tears coursing down her cheeks, stifling any sound with her pillow so as not to disturb Margie. In those midnight hours, she poured out her suffering to God. Unkind remarks that had been made to her—"You must have been cold and unresponsive in your intimate life"; "You must have been difficult to get along with"; "Men don't leave home for no reason at all"; "You probably nagged too much"—sat like stones in her heart.

"God, You know the truth about us. You know none of this makes any sense! Will I ever understand?" she prayed through hot tears.

Her doctor finally insisted that she take sleeping pills, which she did for a while. But the side effects were so devastating that soon she discarded them altogether, claiming the Lord's promises that He would see her through.

At one point Helen made an appointment with an Adventist counselor who had been highly recommended to her. It was a relief to pour out all the pent-up frustration, the agony. She could not believe her ears when he said to her coldly, "Obviously you are lying; you are slanting the truth. If things were as ideal as you say they were, if you and your husband were as much in love as you insist, he would never have gone. Why don't you face the truth?"

In despair, Helen cried, "But I *am* telling the truth! Stan is sick! He is sick!"

With a superior smile, the counselor turned back to his desk. "If it makes you feel better to believe that, who am I to stop you?"

During the last few weeks before Stan left, when Helen finally became aware of his specific plans, she had begged him to write to her and let her know how he was. "Stan," she had sobbed, "you are the dearest person on earth to me. I have to know that you're safe. I have to know that you're all right."

He would not promise. And he did not write to her. Finally a card came—to Margie. Just a few scrawled words from the husband and father who had always written such eloquent, expressive letters. He did not mention Helen. He would not write to Jacquee or to his parents. To Helen's shock, though, on her birthday he sent her a card. His constant contradictions in conduct and action were as mystifying as ever.

The first time a loaded North American Van Lines truck pulled up in front of the little house, Helen was shocked speechless. The man who walked up to the door, wearing work clothes, was not Stan—at least he was not the Stan she had loved and married. He spoke to Helen as though she were a stranger to whom he had just been introduced.

"How is Margie getting along?" he demanded.

"Well, she's doing as well as you could expect under the circumstances," Helen stammered. "All this has been terribly hard on her."

He did not ask for details. He did not ask how she was managing financially. He stayed a day or two, then left. "Who was that stranger?" Helen asked herself, almost disoriented.

During the few brief hours of his visit, Helen saw that his

facial twitchings were as pronounced as ever, that his arms and legs twitched constantly, that his eyes seemed vague and unfocused. She wondered how he had passed his training period at North American Van Lines. Later she would learn that he passed only barely—and this because he was a good driver. Apparently his new employers had had grave misgivings, having become aware, as she was, of his abnormalities.

From time to time he sent small sums of money to Margie. Very small sums. Then, at Christmas, another erratic action—money orders for ten dollars for both Helen and Margie. Helen was thrown off balance. He had apparently rejected them. So what did these little gifts mean?

During her final talk with Stan's doctor at Loma Linda, Helen had told him, "In six months my husband will lose everything financially. He has lost all touch with reality. He doesn't understand anything about money, any more than a child would at this point. He's lost all conception of values. He can't make it alone."

But the doctor did not agree with her.

Six months almost to the day from his departure date, Stan sent Margie a newspaper clipping of his truck, which he had totaled on a highway in the Midwest. Helen would later learn that he had not kept up the insurance on the truck, so it was reclaimed by the company.

But time was working its merciful healing balm in Helen's heart. She became aware gradually that the sky was beginning to seem blue again, that the flowers, always a source of intense joy to her, were as beautiful as they had always been. Food began to have flavor and texture. Margie's friends, full of life, overflowed the little house; Helen felt as comfortable with them as with people her own age—more comfortable, in fact. One day as she was working at her desk in the office, she remembered the words of her doctor when he checked her out of the Glendale Sanitarium: "This isn't the end of the world for you, Helen. You can make a new life for yourself."

Could she do that? Was there still some happiness ahead for her? It began to seem possible.

One day when she came home from work, she found a box from the Mobil Oil Company. "What in the world are they advertising now?" she said to herself. During these months she hadn't been opening her mail each day, for there were so many bills and so many insurance complications and so many disturbing letters from well-meaning acquaintances that someone had suggested she would weather the storm better if she subjected herself to the mail less frequently. Remembering this, she tossed the box into the wastebasket, saying to herself that whatever the Mobil Company was advertising, she wasn't interested. Then some ingrained caution made her go to the wastebasket and pluck the box out. People shouldn't throw mail away unopened, that she knew.

When she saw the stacks and stacks of charge slips in the box, her heart almost stopped. There were gasoline purchases all over the United States, charges for new headlights, new batteries, new tires. The credit card number was correct—it was Stan's card. The total was more than $650, which, for Helen, was an astronomical sum at that point. What should she do? What could she do? Her mind whirling, she sat down. But there was an unknown signature on the slips. Had Stan's card been stolen?

After the wrecking of his truck, Stan had dropped out of sight, not communicating with Margie. Only recently had she received a card from him, telling her he was staying at the Salvation Army hostel in Chicago. Not until long afterward would they learn that after his truck and his job were taken away, and he was penniless, he had loaded potatoes in the bitter Indiana winter, having no place to sleep and no food to eat. He had made his way to Chicago, this pitiful man with a dying mind, and had humbly begged for shelter, which the Salvation Army captain willingly gave.

Immediately Helen wrote to the captain. "Can you please get an explanation from my husband about all these charges?" she begged. "I can't afford to lose my credit, but I haven't the money to pay them, and I'm terrified that more will be coming in."

Again the sleepless nights, the free-floating anxiety. The Salvation Army captain was one of God's people. He understood her panic. He wrote back at once.

"I finally got to the bottom of the credit-card mystery," he told her. "When your husband was loading potatoes in Indiana, he met another man also trying to make some money this way. This man apparently played on his sympathies, saying that if only he could get to Seattle to see his girlfriend and get things straightened out with her, his life would change for the better. Your husband trustingly handed over his credit card, because he was sorry for another man in the same straits he found himself. Of course the man promised that he would mail it back the moment he reached Seattle. Obviously, from what you tell me, he has traveled all over the United States."

Later Helen would find that the unscrupulous man had used the card to secure sums of cash—that some of the purchases listed were only for the purpose of satisfying company regulations in regard to charges. He had found service-station attendants willing to give him the cash he needed.

Helen sat with her head in her hands after reading the captain's letter. Her heart ached for Stan. Poor, poor Stan, always so high-principled himself, so quick to believe the best, so reluctant to see the worst. He had seen another's need and had been a helpless victim of another's machinations.

Though she stopped any further charges on the card immediately, Helen was informed that she would have to pay the $650. After all, the card had not been stolen. It had been used with the knowledge and consent of the owner.

Something in the captain's letter, near the end, puzzled Helen. By now she had become accustomed to—or had accepted—Stan's indifference to her feelings, his lack of concern for what she thought or for what anyone else thought. She knew that on his downhill road he must have given up the Christian life and experience that had been the center of his being. In order to live with this knowledge, she tried to block it out of her mind as far as possible. If he never became the Stan of her young dreams again, then survival for her lay in putting it all behind her. Now a slightly new element entered the picture.

"Your husband is so humiliated, so embarrassed, over this incident. I doubt that he will ever come home now that this has happened. He feels that he has betrayed your trust in him completely." Helen read the words over and over. The letter went on: "I am puzzled by your husband. Mr. Jefferson does not fit the picture of the run-of-the-mill alcoholic or reject of society that usually comes to us. He is a man of refinement and sensitivity. However, he seems to have many physical problems. We tried having him drive one of our trucks, but somehow that didn't work out, and now he is running the freight elevator for us."

When Helen had discovered that Stan was in Chicago, she contacted friends in that area, from Andrews University, Hinsdale Sanitarium, and other places. Would they, could they, spare the time to pay him a brief visit? And they did, one after another. But their report was always the same. He was not the Stan Jefferson they had known; he was remote, unreachable. They all agreed that he would never come home. He would never again be her husband in the full sense of the word.

The possibility that Stan could now be humiliated and embarrassed over his actions and the implication that he was sorry for the way he had treated her surprised Helen after all that had transpired, after all that she had been told.

Feeling that she must have advice following the credit-card incident, Helen counseled with several of her minister friends and others. They were aghast. Almost as one, each said, "Helen, you simply have to have financial protection for yourself and Margie. As long as you and Stan are married, you are responsible for whatever bills he may incur. Sad as it may seem, there is only one safe course open to you—divorce."

The very sound of the word chilled her heart. She was no prude; she had contacted many people in many different situations; she was a realist and knew that divorce was sometimes the only solution to a marriage that was irrevocably broken.

Another friend had said, "Helen, you have so much love to give. You were so loving and warm with Stan. You were meant to be married. You are a very attractive, vital woman. There is absolutely no reason why the Lord shouldn't bring a new love into your life. Think about it."

Helen thought, her blue eyes soft and musing. If only they knew how I long to put my arms around a strong man and have his arms around me. Oh, the inexpressible comfort of a loving relationship! Though she did not speak of it, her physical needs existed; they were unsatisfied. She tried never to think of this phase of her emotional deprivation.

Gradually the realization came to her that she now could put the past behind her. She could accept a new relationship into her life. She could do all these things—if they were God's will. But she had to be absolutely sure that this was the case.

Yet her resolution wavered. "If Stan is sick, as I truly believe he is, then do I have a right to divorce him? Wouldn't that be abandoning him and leaving him with no one?" She asked this question of the lawyer to whom friends had directed her.

"Mrs. Jefferson," he replied, when she had sketched briefly for him the history of Stan's conduct, "it is not up to me to judge whether or not your husband is ill. Perhaps he is. I can only say that in California you are responsible for all the bills as long as you are married. I can send letters of notification to every place you think he might charge, but that is only a flimsy protection at best. Perhaps if he is indeed as sick as you say, it is imperative that you file for divorce as soon as possible, since you have no way of knowing what he will do. Your daughter deserves this protection."

Margie. Just how she was paying Margie's school bills Helen could not tell. Week by week, month by month, somehow the bills were being paid. Looking back in later years, Helen would feel that the Lord had worked financial miracles, that the dollars she had been given contained two hundred cents, not one hundred. Moreover, her status as an employee was so cloudy that she received almost none of the benefits that many other women employees received. She was not single; she did not qualify for head-of-the-house benefits. But she was not married, either. Sometimes, hearing other secretaries speaking of the generous allowances they were given for various purposes, her heart burned within her. She was ashamed of her feelings, but it so frequently seemed that fair play was never taken into account. "The policy says . . ." became the nemesis of her life.

In view of all this, and realizing that once a divorce took place she could be given more benefits that would help Margie, Helen at last came to the decision. She would institute proceedings for the divorce. But she wanted to make one last test, one last request of the Lord. On the Friday night after she had made the decision, she was invited to attend an It Is Written meeting in Long Beach. When Elder George Vandeman made an altar call, both for those who wished to accept Christ for the first time and for those who wished a closer experience with Christ, Helen went forward. With hot tears coursing down her cheeks, she pleaded with the Lord. "Show me what I ought to do, dear Jesus," she said to herself. "If he is as sick as I think he is, do I have the right to abandon him? But I'm so tired, Lord, and I need a new beginning so badly. Please don't let me make a mistake. Please make it perfectly clear to me what I ought to do."

The answer came two weeks later.

Stan wrote her a letter. "Can you ever forgive me and take me back?" was the message in every line. She could not believe her eyes. The words swam in front of her. Only a few short weeks before, the Salvation Army captain had written that he was sure Stan would never return home, never resume his life with Helen and his family and friends. Helen thought with what unbounded joy she would have received Stan's letters last July, August, September. Now she had reached the point of considering a new life for herself, of throwing off the burden of Stan's illness, his intransigence, the hopelessness of it all. She had begun to have moments when she felt light and free and young. Even as those thoughts crossed her mind, she dismissed them as unworthy.

In her room alone, with thoughts too deep for tears, she wondered, if she did not forgive Stan, how she could ever sincerely pray those beautiful words, "Forgive us our debts, as we forgive our debtors." With the oneness the two of them had shared, she knew that in his weak condition he had run from hurts he could not endure, from problems he was incapable of facing. Dropping to her knees, she said, simply, "Dear Lord, I accept Your answer to my plea for guidance. I will tell Stan to come home."

When Margie came in from class, instantly she sensed that something was different. "What is it, Mother?" she asked fearfully, herself now as apprehensive as Helen was, wondering what new development would take place from day to day.

"Daddy wants to come back to us," Helen told her, and her blue eyes filled with tears. Tears of joy?

Margie was ecstatic. "Oh, I'm so glad, so glad, so glad. I just knew he wouldn't stay away from us," she cried, hugging Helen. "Daddy loves us too much not to be with us."

"Stan dear," Helen wrote to him, "come home—right

now. Today, the fastest way you can come. If you need money, I'll send it to you. Margie and I will be counting the minutes."

But there was a problem. He would not let her pay his way home. His pride had suffered too keenly. "I will pay my own way home," he wrote, "and it will take me a little while to earn it."

Helen wisely understood.

And so early in May, Helen and Margie went to the bus station to meet him. Helen's breath caught in her throat at the sight of him. He was so thin as to be almost emaciated. The good clothes he had had when he left—and Stan had always been a fastidious dresser—were gone, where she did not know. He was wearing an ill-fitting tweed suit that he proudly told her he had gotten at the Salvation Army. "I wanted to look nice for you," he said shyly.

As the two of them hugged him, Helen noticed, with a sinking heart, that his facial grimaces were much, much worse, that the twitching in his arms and legs was more pronounced, that the contours of his face seemed somewhat changed, almost blurred. He was deteriorating inexorably. At that moment Helen made her decision. She would never leave Stan, never forsake him. In that blinding flash of understanding she came to believe that all the sorrows and trials of her young life with her invalid mother had prepared her for this responsibility. "God needed someone for Stan who would take care of him no matter what," she said to herself. "I am that person. I know what it means to have life disrupted by illness. The Lord will help me cope."

Mercifully, she could not know what would be involved in her dedication. She could not know what would be required of her in the long years ahead.

CHAPTER 13
The End of Hoping

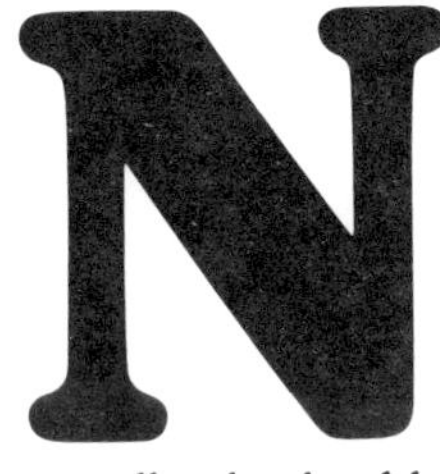

OW a different life began, a life that seemed out of focus, strange, and temporary. Helen got up each morning at the ring of the alarm clock (though usually she had been awake for some time), fixed breakfast for the three of them, and hurried to her office. Margie went to the hospital, to her classes and clinics. And Stan? Stan sat endlessly in the house, his arms and legs twitching, his face contorted, his mind clouded. He communicated with the two of them very little, though at times he made brief comments on his life away from them. They never learned all that had transpired. Actually, the subject was too painful to think and talk about. At times he was impatient, irritable, moody.

Even on that first Friday night, so strained, so unreal, there could not be the peace and tranquillity for which Helen so longed. Stan's jaw had been throbbing all day; the pain became excruciating. He was unable to cope with the agony. Hastily Helen phoned a dentist friend.

"I think Stan has an abscessed tooth," she faltered, "and I hate to ask you on Friday night, but we really need help."

The dentist didn't fail her. At his office he took temporary measures to relieve the pain, then extensive dental work ensued—not only extensive, but expensive. On her limited income, every medical or dental emergency was terrifying to Helen.

"I can't go on like this!" Stan burst out one day. "I have to work. I have to have a job like other men."

Helen realized his humiliation. But what could he do? How could he function as an employee?

"Stan," she told him, "first let's see another doctor and

perhaps now we can find out something that will make you feel better."

He was willing. He was always willing to attempt anything that would relieve him of his torment, torment that he seemed unable to put into words. Marvin, Helen's brother, recommended a well-known brain surgeon, who agreed to see Stan as soon as possible. After the examination, he came into the office where Helen was waiting, his face grave.

"Mrs. Jefferson," he said, "I am very much afraid your husband has Huntington's disease or encephalitis damage. If so, the future is going to be a lot harder on you than on him. But I want another doctor to examine him, to make sure of my diagnosis."

Between the two appointments, Helen was sleepless.

The second doctor confirmed the diagnosis. Stan was a victim of Huntington's chorea. The long, sad saga had come to a turning point. Her steadfast declaration that Stan was incurably sick had been proved correct. Now there was an explanation for so much that had mystified her. Now she need no longer feel rejected. He was not responsible for what he had done. He could not help it.

"Mrs. Jefferson," the second doctor told her, "I cannot tell you how important it is for you to know what you are facing. I can think of no disease more tragic for a patient and his family than H.D. I am going to give you some literature to read, so that you will know—at least in part—what to expect. But there really is no way to put into words the tragedy of the gradual deterioration of both mind and body that takes place. The patient becomes a stranger in his personal habits, his outlook, and his actions. There is really no humiliation that a sufferer of H.D. does not undergo. One part of the tragedy is that while the patient seems to understand, at least at first, that he is very ill, the frontal lobes of his brain are so affected that his judgment is soon completely gone. His irrational actions appear to him perfectly normal. It is as though he is a creature from another planet, a lower order of being set down among superior beings and yet must cope. The disease is not fatal; usually pneumonia or heart complications finally are the immediate cause of death. How merciful if the end could be more swift!"

When Helen began to read some of the material the doctor had given her, she had to put it aside for a day or two, praying for both strength and composure. The brutal phrases leaped out at her—"chronic, progressive, and degenerative disease of the central nervous system." When the articles went on to describe the deterioration of the patient, the lack of bowel and bladder control that would develop, the constant jerking and twitching of all the muscles, the loss of judgment and finally sanity itself, Helen threw herself on her knees beside her bed. Her heart was too heavy for conscious words to form. She could only say, over and over, "Lord, help us. Lord, help us."

Would Stan, her fastidious, immaculate Stan, courteous, refined, considerate, sink to the animal level? Surely he would live and suffer only three or four years at the most. She could not know that his torture—and hers—would last for sixteen years.

"I must face it one day at a time," she told herself, trying to push back the panic that almost overwhelmed her. "God's grace is sufficient. He will not forsake me, and I know I will be given wisdom for the decisions I will have to make."

Then there was the sad task of telling Margie, who had surmised the truth, and Jacquee, and the two sets of parents. The latter were stricken, were almost speechless. They had agonized over Stan's betrayal of Helen and his girls, but this was, in its way, infinitely worse.

"Isn't there any—cure?" Helen's mother faltered.

"None," Helen told her sorrowfully.

Stan's parents could hardly comprehend, could hardly accept, the verdict. They hoped against hope. Surely the diagnosis was in error; surely something new would come to light; surely . . .

But life must be coped with on an everyday basis. Both doctors had told Helen that as long as Stan felt able to work, he should be given a simple, comprehensible job that would not be beyond his capabilities and would not put too much stress on his deteriorating mind and body. A friend of Helen's hesitantly suggested that housekeeping help was badly needed at the hospital.

"Do you think Stan could fit into that?" she asked hesitantly.

Helen thanked her, grateful for the suggestion. Stan's return had caused a great lifting of eyebrows in many quarters. She was all too aware that some people felt he had had his fling, and now, tired of it, had returned to Helen. They were not prepared to accept the fact that he was ill. Others, though, were deeply compassionate, and Helen grasped their proffered love and understanding eagerly.

When Stan applied at the hospital for custodial work and was accepted, he was very happy, very proud. "I'm going to be bringing in money again and that will ease the load on you," he told Helen, much as he would have done in their young years. He did not seem to grasp the difference between being a minister and being in custodial work. She was grateful for this.

"I'm going to do everything I can to improve my health," he also resolved. He took walks, daily, miles and miles. He exercised on a regular routine, including push-ups. He was aware that he had been diagnosed as having Huntington's disease, but his weakened mind seemed not to grasp the full implications, which Helen thought was merciful.

His work at the hospital was very satisfactory. Enough of the old Stan remained to make him meticulous in the performance of his duties. As time passed, he was actually supervising the other men in the custodial department.

"I'd like to put Stan in as head of the household department," one of the administrators told Helen after several months.

Helen did not answer at once. Then she said, "I don't think he could stand the strain. His judgment is impaired, you know, by his disease, and it seems best for him not to be put to any great stress, but I do appreciate your interest in him."

Helen discovered by accident one of the most poignant episodes in Stan's now-pitiful life. When he arrived home one late afternoon, she saw traces of tears on his cheeks.

"What's the matter, dear?" she asked gently.

"I walked to the house we built on Vallejo Drive and looked at it," he told her chokingly.

She put her arms around him silently. As the months passed she knew that the scene repeated itself from time to time. She wondered what thoughts were in his troubled mind as he looked at the house they had planned and built so lovingly. Did he wonder what might have been? As the slow tears coursed down his cheeks did he understand the magnitude of his tragedy?

Margie had reestablished her old, sweet relationship with her father. He responded to her love as to no one else. Jacquee phoned frequently. Both sets of parents made clear their love and support. But Helen knew that Stan must fight yet another battle. He would never feel comfortable in his home again, would never feel secure in his life with her unless he made his peace with God. An inspiration came. A college friend, now Elder Douglas Marchus, was the chaplain of Glendale Adventist Hospital, where Stan did custodial work. Doug and Stan had actually roomed together one year at PUC. Doug would understand, she was sure, and moreover, he would be willing to help.

"Doug," she told him when she had made the appointment to talk with him in his office, "Stan needs the help that probably only you can give. Before his mind deteriorates further, he needs to make his peace with God. I know that he cannot be even partially relaxed until this takes place. Will you help?"

"In every way I can" was Doug's response. He

proceeded to create opportunities for the two of them to meet and to talk. Slowly and carefully he carried Stan back through the years, and they analyzed what had happened. Helen would never know all that Stan told Doug, and she did not want to know. It was with a feeling of unutterable gratitude that one day she heard Stan say to her, "Snooksie, I want to be rebaptized. I know that I have wandered far away from God, and I know that I have let Him down and let others down and turned my back on all that is right. But I believe that God is willing to forgive me."

"I know He is!" Helen exclaimed, her blue eyes swimming with tears. "You can't know how wonderful this is—how happy it makes me, Stan." In Helen's heart God had worked a small miracle. She was free of any feeling of resentment for what might have transpired when Stan was away from home. He was in despair. He had been told that he was not sick. He was confused, did not know where to turn. If he had known that he was incurably sick, he would never have left home, never have left the sheltering arms of those who loved him.

They knelt together and she prayed. After a moment of hesitation, Stan prayed, a stumbling prayer of only a few words. But it was enough for Helen. She knew that in his now-limited way he was going as far as he could.

Stan told Doug that he felt he must do more than enter into rebaptism. "I have set such a terrible example," he said. "I want to make a public statement and hope that it will repair some of the damage I have done."

Doug was willing. Helen was filled with trepidation. She wondered what he would say. She wondered whether he would be an object of ridicule, if his contorted face and twitching limbs would cause others to look down on him. She hoped that he would mention his illness, would make it clear that he had not fully understood what he had done and probably never would. But he said nothing of this.

"I looked at the mistakes and sins of others and became

discouraged," he said simply. "I confess that I have shamed my Saviour. Today I want to renew my commitment to Him and show by my rebaptism that I love and serve Him."

For one brief, shining moment, as Stan stood at the pulpit, it seemed to Helen that he was her own dear, loving, handsome, young Stan—the evangelist of her dreams, leading his congregations. Then the moment passed.

Though his baptism seemed to comfort him, Stan never again seemed able to concentrate long enough to study his Bible for any length of time. His mind, impaired as it was, could feed on only superficial material. But Helen was comforted by her conviction that the Lord knew what Stan could and couldn't do, and accepted His flawed human child just as he was.

When, after Stan had been away for several months, Helen had received word that his ministerial credentials had been revoked, she had thought that her heart, by now used to hammer blows, could not survive this one. Stan was a *minister.* That was his life. That was her life. He had been consecrated, had been set apart for life. Yet she knew she must be fair and reasonable. She thought to herself, If this were some other minister, would I feel that it was fair to remove his credentials, in view of his conduct? The sorrowful answer came back, Yes. But she continued to pray that sometime, someday, the credentials would be restored. How, she did not know. It was a hope that never left her. But it was never to be.

Helen's devotional reading assumed greater and greater importance in her life as the magnitude of the tragedy became clearer. One day, while reading *Steps to Christ*, she came upon a paragraph that she copied and virtually memorized during the next years!

> The assurance is broad and unlimited, and He is faithful who has promised. When we do not receive the very things we asked for, at the time we ask, we are still to believe that the Lord hears, and that He will answer our

> prayers. We are so erring and shortsighted that we sometimes ask for things that would not be a blessing to us, and our heavenly Father in love answers our prayers by giving us that which will be for our highest good—that which we ourselves would desire if with vision divinely enlightened we could see all things as they really are. When our prayers seem not to be answered, we are to cling to the promise; for the time of answering will surely come, and we shall receive the blessing we need most. But to claim that prayer will always be answered in the very way and for the particular thing that we desire, is presumption. God is too wise to err, and too good to withhold any good thing from them that walk uprightly. Then do not fear to trust Him, even though you do not see the immediate answer to your prayers. Rely upon His sure promise, "Ask, and it shall be given you."—Page 96.

Like a flash of blinding light, Helen's mind was again illuminated. The thing she had wrestled with for so long—her prayers before her marriage, her request that she not have illness in her home—became clearer. Even though she had thought in the past that she had understood, she had not. Could it be that God wanted someone to care for Stan with the love and compassion that she was able to give? In His wisdom, did God consider her capable of this assignment because of the years she had spent in the crucible of self-sacrifice during her childhood and youth? From then on, she was seldom troubled by the devil's questions on this point.

Helen became aware that the Lord was working another miracle in her heart. By now she was reading all the material she could find on Huntington's disease. She visited medical libraries, the public library—she consulted medical friends. Everything she read and heard emphasized over and over that a victim of Huntington's disease becomes a repugnant creature, unacceptable even to those who have loved him deeply before he was stricken.

But as the days and weeks and months, and then years, passed, Helen found that the Lord was taking from her heart all negative emotions toward Stan, leaving it full of pity and compassion. No matter how unreasonable he became in later years, she still loved him. She took what came, day by day. Sometimes, when he had been particularly unreasonable (even at times using words that were never part of the old Stan's vocabulary), she did not reply in kind.

Stan could not know that sometimes when she had gone to her office, as she sat at her desk the tears would come and she would wipe them away hastily, hoping that no one had seen.

But there were still internal struggles for Helen, brought on at times by the knowledge that ministers of her acquaintance who suffered severe illnesses were able to retain their credentials, to be given financial assistance, and in general to retain their position in the sight of their peers.

"If only Stan had been diagnosed in time" was a refrain that beat through her thoughts for years of sad days. Yet to hold bitterness in her heart on that account was, she realized, to negate all that God was trying to do for her in the area of accepting what she could not change. "I don't mind so much for myself, Father," she prayed, "but it breaks my heart that Stan has been disgraced and that what should have been regarded as illness was thought of by everyone as repudiation of You." Sometimes she thought she had achieved victory over her feelings. At other times she knew that she had not.

One of the hardest and most frightening aspects of life for Helen was the necessity for her to make all the decisions, financial and otherwise. She had no one to whom she felt she could turn for counsel, with the exception of her brother. But she dreaded loading her problems on others.

"Mother," Margie burst out one day, "what am I going to do? I will have to move back to Loma Linda for my public-health affiliation in San Bernardino. I just don't see how I can manage without a car."

Helen felt her heart begin to beat faster, as it always did when a new and apparently insoluble problem presented itself. They were barely scraping by financially. How could they manage another car?

"Margie, the Lord knows our needs. He hasn't forsaken us thus far, and He won't forsake us now. We'll get another car, one way or another."

Taking her courage in her hands, Helen spoke to one or two of the conference officers. They were sympathetic and helpful.

"There's no use in your getting a car that will give you nothing but problems," she was told. "You need good, reliable transportation. Have you thought of seeing what price a dealer would make you on a demonstrator?"

Helen hadn't thought of that, but she acted on the suggestion at once. First, though, she had to appear to include Stan. He still felt that he should be a part of the decision-making process, that he should be consulted, especially in the area of cars, certainly his province, or so he thought. His driving had become so erratic and so unreliable that Helen was terrified to have him at the wheel. Yet he insisted on driving.

"Let's go and look at cars!" Helen exclaimed brightly, and after much tact on her part, and the obvious understanding of a friendly dealer, a demonstrator was found that just fit the bill.

When she was told suddenly that she would have to vacate the tiny house that she and Margie had fixed up so lovingly, Helen became convinced that she was one of the devil's special targets. "Now don't be such an egotist!" she scolded herself. "Do you think you're so important that the devil would lie awake nights figuring out every possible trial for you?" She had to smile at the mental picture this conjured up, but still— And when the only thing she could find to move into that she could afford was a small, very dark, very damp apartment, she wondered even more about her status in the devil's book of trials.

As she struggled with the moving, Stan and Margie helping as best they could, Helen had to go into the bathroom and wipe away surreptitious tears. She and Stan had started out in a tent with nothing. They had never had any help through the bitterly hard years. With frugality beyond belief, they had gradually acquired their first tiny home, then another a bit better, then another, until there had been the new house in Glendale that they had lived in so briefly, and then the pretty home in Oakland—and then it had been downhill all the way. Now all their equity was gone. Stan's profession was gone. They were almost back to where they had started.

But not quite. There were Jacquee and Margie and the happy memories of the good years.

"Please help me not to give in to discouragement," Helen prayed. And swiftly her mood lightened. Perhaps there were still some good days ahead, sometime, somewhere.

Stan insisted on continuing to drive the car, a circumstance that terrified both Helen and Margie. After each foray onto the crowded freeways with Stan, Helen would come back limp and drained.

"Stan," she tried to reason with him, "you take such chances. You change lanes so abruptly. You don't signal. You exceed the speed limit."

"I'm as good a driver as anyone else!" he shouted at her. "I've driven all my life, and I'm not stopping now!"

And he didn't. The terror on the freeways continued.

Now Helen, who never gave up hoping that something could be done for Stan to arrest the course of his disease, made an appointment with a prominent psychiatrist who had been highly recommended. The latter was careful, thorough, meticulous in his evaluation, through several sessions in his office. At last he asked Helen to come for the results of the tests. She could see that he was reluctant to begin the conversation. In his eyes she read deep compassion.

"Mrs. Jefferson," he finally began, gently, "I wish there were an easier way to tell you this, but it would be unfair for me to tell you that your husband can ever be stabilized or that he can be helped. His condition is very serious."

"Are you telling me that it is really hopeless?" Helen faltered.

"Yes—it is hopeless," he replied softly.

As Helen walked down the stairs to the outdoors, each step she took seemed to repeat the refrain, "Hopeless—hopeless—hopeless." She had counted so on this doctor's opinion. Where could she now turn?

"You see," she had said to the doctor, "the problem comes on the everyday level in living with what appears to be two different people. At times Stan seems like his old self—capable, calm, in command of the situation. Then in the twinkling of an eye, he's irresponsible, unstable, out of control, saying strange things and doing incredible things."

"I know" had been the doctor's reply. "That's the terrible part of H.D. That's why the loved ones of a victim are in such torture."

Three weeks later Helen experienced another aspect of the cruelty of this world. Her mother was killed in an automobile accident in Reno.

"No! No—it can't be!" was her reaction when the phone call came. "I can't give up my mother; I can't!"

Everything seemed blurred. The accident itself, outside of Reno, so unnecessary and so final. The arrangements for her and Stan to go to Reno (Margie could not go; she had heavy tests that had to be taken). Jacquee meeting them in Reno, wept.

"Jacquee, you loved your grandmother, didn't you?" Helen asked the red-haired young woman.

"More than almost anyone in the world!" Jacquee sobbed.

Even the funeral rubbed on Helen's raw nerves and heart, for it had been a family decision that the casket would not be opened. Helen had not seen her mother. But Jacquee, strong-minded as ever, would not leave things in this unsatisfactory way. She had loved her grandmother with all the intensity of her nature. After the funeral, when everyone had left the chapel, she stormed up to the funeral director.

"You are not going to bury my grandmother without my having at least looked at her," she told him. "I want you to open her casket at once."

Startled, he agreed, not realizing that there had been a difference of opinion in the family.

As soon as she glimpsed her grandmother, Jacquee said, "Wait here. Keep the casket open." Then she went flying outdoors, where Helen was already sitting alone in the limousine.

"Mother, come back and see Grandma," she begged. "She looks so sweet. You will feel so much better after you have seen her."

Weak-kneed, Helen followed Jacquee, and the two of them stood together at the casket.

"Oh, thank you, Jacquee," Helen told her daughter tremblingly. "Grandma's face is a little swollen, and that actually makes her look more like she did when I was a little girl. I am so glad—so glad—you made it possible for me to see her." But Helen could not cry. She was numb from all her hurts, all her tragedies.

After they returned to California, though, Jacquee had a recurring nightmare for six months. She would dream that she was sitting by Grandma's rocker and that Grandma was reading to her, as she did when Jacquee was a child. In her dream she saw a bay window with a casket in its aperture. Grandma would get out of the casket, sit in the chair, read to Jacquee, then get back in the casket and pull the lid down.

When the nightmares first began, Jacquee phoned Helen

in horror. "I can't live with these dreams," she told her. "It is so utterly real and so horrifying that when I wake up I'm bathed in perspiration and shaking from head to foot."

Alarmed for Jacquee's sensitive nervous system, Helen made suggestion after suggestion. A tepid bath before retiring. Warm milk. Half an hour of reading the Bible or the inspirational books of Ellen White. Prayer. Finally the dreams ceased, but not before Helen's own nerves were strained to the breaking point in both sympathy and dread for Jacquee.

Another heartbreak for Helen to cope with was her father, once so strong, so cheerful, so much the leader of his family. Now he was old, broken in spirit.

"They wouldn't even let me go to my darling's funeral," he sobbed to Helen when she had visited him in the hospital at Reno.

"But, Daddy, they thought your injuries were too serious," she soothed him. "They didn't think you could do it."

"But they had no right to make that decision," he cried bitterly.

And as his bitterness and lack of resignation deepened as time passed, Helen would come to feel that it had indeed been a mistake.

As soon as he was well enough to travel, Helen had brought him to her little apartment in Glendale, since that was what he begged to do. "Please let me live with you and Stan," he begged over and over.

Helen was deeply troubled. How could she turn her back on her father, who needed her so badly? Yet how could she cope with both him and Stan in the small, dark apartment where none of them could have any privacy? And was it fair for Margie, still so young, to live in this atmosphere of sorrow?

On the latter question, she came to a decision, hard though it was.

"Margie, my dear," she told the petite, gentle girl, "I know you must move into the dormitory at Loma Linda while you are taking your last year of nursing. I don't think you should come home every weekend. You are young and all your life is ahead of you. The situation here is just too negative at the moment, and I will feel better if you're not so involved. Spend as many weekends with your friends out there as possible."

Loyal little Margie, though, came home often, lifting her mother's load. After she graduated, Helen advised that she share an apartment with a friend.

"Mommy, I just don't see how we're going to pay my tuition clear through to the end," Margie had worried from time to time. "You don't get the educational allowance you got when Daddy was a minister. Maybe I should drop out and get a job——"

Helen would never let her continue.

"You're going to get your nursing degree," she always replied sturdily. "I don't know how, but it's going to happen."

It did happen, and Helen was right. When Margie went down the aisle on graduation day, the bill was *paid*. Looking back through the years, she would never know where the money came from. When she simply had to have it, it came. Helen and Margie never lost their sense of humor. "Mom," Margie said to her one day, "do you realize what a great career you could have had as Secretary of the Treasury of the United States?"

"Well, I'm willing any time they are," Helen chuckled. "On the other hand, maybe I'd better look for a job in the circus as a juggler—I'm so used to juggling the bills and keeping everything from crashing to the ground!"

Margie's enormous stability was something Helen thanked God for every night. This petite, fragile girl never seemed to run out of love and understanding for her father and grandfather. She never seemed to think of herself, and never did Helen hear Margie say that she resented the tragedy that had come to their family. She just went on her loving way, like a little cricket on the hearth.

But the situation with Helen's father continued to deteriorate. When she left him in the mornings to go to the office, he would weep.

"I'm so lonesome. I miss your mother so much," he told her.

Helen would sit at her desk, wondering how she could calm her troubled thoughts and give her full time and attention to her job so as to turn out the kind of excellent work that was her hallmark. When she would race home at noon to fix lunch, her father would meet her at the door, crying. When she returned home at the end of her day's work, he would cry.

Stan's deterioration continued. The twitching never stopped. His outbursts continued from time to time. The reckless driving got worse. His mind was at times vague and unfocused. But he continued to go to his janitorial job, and the only bright spot of that particular period was that finally he was able to clear off the $650 that had been charged to his credit card by his "friend." Helen felt lighter, as though a load had been taken from her shoulders. Stan had doggedly kept at it until the bill was completely cleared away.

In a reversion to what he had once been, Stan hugged her. "Snooksie, I know how that debt has worried you, and I'm so glad it's paid," he declared.

Finally Helen had to admit defeat so far as her father was concerned; she had to take him back to Reno. Others could take care of him, but only she could take care of Stan.

Helen had been told by the doctors that Stan would live fifteen or twenty years or more, going downhill until one day he would have to be institutionalized. The very word sent panic racing through her body. Must he eventually be placed in a State institution where he would receive care—but not the kind a loving family could provide? How could she pay for private care? What would she do?

When these thoughts beat through her brain during

sleepless nights, she begged for relief. Prayer was her only solace. Occasionally she would feel like a drowning person going under. Then a beautiful Bible verse would flash into her tired mind—"Fear thou not; for I am with thee"—and there would be a temporary lessening of the fear and apprehension. Sometimes she would hear the devil telling her she really couldn't claim to be a child of God since she had so little faith and trust in Him. She would weep with remorse and a feeling of guilt.

During the day, though, she had to keep up a cheerful, steady attitude for Stan. He seemed to sense her inner turmoil at times, and at this stage of his illness would still put his arms around her and try to comfort her in his dazed, uncomprehending way, knowing that something was wrong but not really able to grasp the magnitude of what was happening.

She longed for a human confidant to pour out all her troubles and heartaches to. But her brothers had troubles of their own. Margie, closest to her, was the one she wished above all to protect from permanent scarring. Jacquee's marital troubles had reached a new crescendo, this in itself sending Helen further down the road of depression. As she saw Jacquee struggling with monumental debts, and at one point actually having to put her little boy into a foster home because she herself could not take proper care of him, Helen wondered how many times a heart can break and still go on beating.

Through the years of Stan's ministry Helen had become accustomed to the rather rich social life of a minister's wife. She had enjoyed the contacts with others to the full; she loved people. Outgoing and sociable by nature, she reveled in the Saturday-night socials; she looked forward to the Sabbath dinners when she entertained as many as twelve or fourteen guests. She felt a warm glow of "belonging" at workers' meetings and other church gatherings when she and Stan lunched and dined with other ministerial couples.

She had, she realized, almost taken the frequent invitations for granted.

Now it was all changed.

In the Seventh-day Adventist Church, as in all religious groups, there was an unwritten law—a code. A minister who "went wrong" was in disgrace. Not only he but all the members of his family were subtly "included out." Now there were no more invitations. None of the ministerial couples they had been so close to in the past invited them to spend an evening or attend a concert. The phone did not ring. When Helen took Stan to church each Sabbath, as she had resolved to do for as long as possible, she was painfully aware of the averted glances, the whispers.

"Oh, please don't!" she wanted to shout. "I'm just the same as I've always been. And Stan is sick—so sick. Can't you see that, and can't you be kind? Can't you love us even if we aren't worthy of your love?"

But of course the words were never said.

Helen didn't give up without a struggle. She tried inviting one couple at a time for Sabbath dinner; the apartment was too tiny for any more. But Stan went into panic. He could not converse; could not seem to relate to his duties as a host. Sadly Helen concluded that unless she could invite a group, it just wouldn't work. And since she couldn't do that, perhaps for the time being, the social life would have to lie dormant. When finally this bitter realization came to her, slow tears coursed down her cheeks. After the years of isolation in junior and senior high and the hard years in Salt Lake City, she needed people.

"The Lord knows all about my needs," she told herself, wiping the unbidden tears away. "He'll supply something in place of social life."

And He did. Suddenly it dawned on her that by reading and studying the beautiful and true, she could associate with the Ruler of the heavens and the heavenly hosts. Now the time she spent with the Bible and the Spirit of Prophecy books was more precious than ever. It was part of her "social life."

Her plants, always a great source of satisfaction, now became her "friends." They fitted into her resolve to study the beautiful of life. "Moreover," she said to herself, "I can choose to dress as nicely as possible on my little income, and I'm going to dress Stan just as well as it is possible for me to do. Perhaps the deterioration won't be so noticeable to others so quickly when he is well-dressed."

On one happy day Helen suddenly prayed, "Lord, I'm turning my bank book over to You. I'll follow Your leading every step of the way, and I'll live in any way You show me."

What a load of worry slid off her shoulders at that decision!

There were other rays of light that penetrated the darkness that Stan's illness cast about their lives. Medical research was beginning to discover preparations that helped some of the intense facial grimaces and muscle spasms. When this was prescibed for Stan, he experienced enough relief to bring some joy to Helen's landscape. Sometimes the medication was more effective than other times; yet without it she knew he would have become much worse.

It was always difficult for Stan to accept the necessity for his medications. Earlier in his life, he had taken no medications of any sort, not even aspirin, believing that the body would heal itself if given proper care. But when he was without his medications, he could easily wear the skin off any part of his body that was in constant contact with surfaces.

All her life Helen had wanted to paint, from her childhood through the school year when she was asked to join the art class but felt that her father could not buy her the necessary supplies. All her life she had loved hand-painted china. Suddenly she discovered that near the apartment lived a china-painting teacher who did beautiful work. Helen gathered up her courage one day, phoned, and asked the price of lessons. When she heard the estimate, she thought,

Why, I can afford that! And even though she discovered, as the months passed, that the teacher's estimate had been decidedly low, still she continued. Her pretty china dishes became new "friends."

One day Helen began to feel very sick, very strange. "My chest feels so heavy," she told Stan, though she seldom told him anything negative, lest his twitching and near-convulsions become worse. But she was apprehensive about herself, and so she went to her doctor that day. He told her she had pneumonia. Margie came rushing home.

"You have a built-in nurse, Mom," the little redhead assured her. "Now you must relax and I'm going to take care of you."

"But what about your father, and my job, and—" Helen wept.

"All in good time" was Margie's response. "You just take your medicine, and cuddle down in bed, and *heal!*"

But it was six months before Helen felt really strong again, even though in a short time she began dragging herself to the office.

Her emotional condition became somewhat precarious, probably as the result of her illness, but undoubtedly it was more directly traceable to the continual strain under which she lived. There was never a waking moment when she could feel lighthearted about Stan, knowing so well what the future would bring. On top of this, family members who were having problems came to Helen both for sympathy and counsel. Then Helen had taken on the responsibility of nursery-school payments for Jacquee's children, though Jacquee had not asked her to do this. Her mind ached with all her thoughts. How could she be "all things to all people"?

Finally she made a decision. She would see a psychiatrist. Was it natural to feel so depressed and beaten? Until now, she had thought that only seriously disturbed people visited psychiatrists, but she was desperate. She had heard good things about a doctor in San Marino. Her visit to his office marked a turning point in her life. After she had explained to him her responsibilities, all her loads, he said quietly, "You don't have a serious mental or emotional problem. In fact, you are unusually strong and stable. I doubt that very many people could take all you have taken and still function."

He paused, then went on firmly, "But you will not be able to continue unless you assimilate a great truth right now. You are not in this world to solve all the problems of those you love. I grant that your husband has no one else. But as for the others—they will have to find other solutions. You cannot go on being the solution to so many problems. If you follow my counsel, you will, I am confident, survive, and survive well."

When Helen went home and prayed about the doctor's counsel, she felt impressed that he was right and that she had been led to see him. She resolved to take a no-nonsense approach to life, to do only what she could, and leave the rest to the Lord.

"After all," she said to herself with a smile, "nobody has appointed me vice-president of the universe!"

CHAPTER 14
Doing What Must Be Done

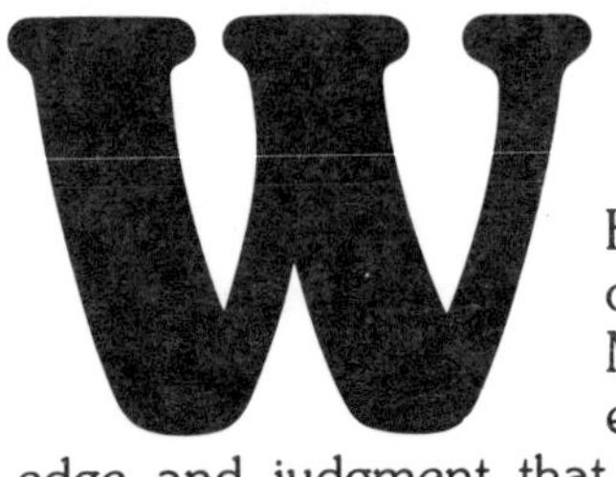

HEN Helen turned her finances over to the Lord as her "General Manager," she knew that He expected her to use the knowledge and judgment that she had acquired through her lifetime. A source of great concern to her was that she and Stan had lost the equity in their homes and were now without any security for the future. Because of his indeterminate condition for the year he was away, she had not been given the maximum benefits that would have been so helpful to her. She knew that before long Stan would require more care than she could give him. She was making rather large car payments. The two of them were living in the little dark apartment. They owned nothing.

"If I could just buy a little piece of land—just a little piece," Helen whispered to herself. But how could she? She couldn't travel around the State of California looking for a tiny plot that she could afford. But her astute financial sense kept reminding her that probably her only chance of establishing some security was in buying land and letting it appreciate. She began to pray about this almost obsessively.

Helen shared an office with another secretary whose husband was one of the publishing directors. One morning her friend said, rather idly, "Would you believe it? There are ten acres of land we've been trying to buy for a long time and now that we've moved here to Glendale and bought a house and can't afford the acreage, we've gotten a letter telling us the owners would like to sell!"

Instantly Helen was interested. "Tell me all about it!" she begged.

"Well," said her friend, "it really is beautiful land with beautiful timber. It's on the shores of a tiny lake—a man-made lake, but a lake nevertheless."

Helen found that her heart was beating fast. By the most careful planning and watching every penny, she had managed to save seven hundred dollars. She got an idea.

"Do you think you and your husband could swing five acres?" she asked hopefully.

Her friend thought for a moment. "Why, yes, I think we could."

"If you make the arrangements for the ten acres, then I'll buy five acres from you," was Helen's offer. "This is just an answer to prayer. I know you'll tell me that you don't want me to buy land sight unseen and ordinarily I would agree, but you are one of my very best friends and I believe you and trust you. If you think it's a good investment for you, it will be a good investment for me."

Finally all the arrangements were made. Helen paid $500 as a down payment, with monthly payments to be settled later. Taxes on the property were only twenty or twenty-five dollars a year. Finally, two years later, the road was all laid and the surveys completed, and Helen found that some of her land would be under water, so the price was lowered to $4,000 and the payments to thirty-five dollars.

This first attempt to recoup some of her financial losses was a great lift to her spirits. Her land was situated about thirty miles south of Sonora, in the foothills 3,500 feet in altitude.

A bright spot in Helen's life was the double wedding of Margie and Jacquee in Sacramento. Jacquee had worked her way through the massive problems surrounding her first marriage. She had managed to pay off the debts and secure a divorce. She had met a fine man, a lawyer. Margie had become engaged to a young Seventh-day Adventist man who was exactly what Helen had hoped Margie would find.

"We're going to have a double wedding in Sacramento," they told her.

Pleased as she was at the news, Helen's blue eyes filled with tears. "I wish I could afford to give you a nice wedding," she told them, "but you know that is impossible."

They were quick to reassure her. "Don't you worry. We're each going to wear a light suit and a little hat with a veil. We'll look just great and it will be nice."

It *was* nice. Only the families of the brides and grooms attended. Helen, sitting on the front row, found a small lump in her throat. How she used to dream of beautiful church weddings for her two pretty red-haired daughters! But she quickly told herself that superficial things did not matter. The fact of the love each had found was what was important.

Stan attended the wedding and seemed at times almost like his old self. Again she wondered, How can this horror be true? He was so kind and loving with Jacquee's children. They seemed to understand that something was flawed in him, but gave him their total acceptance. He was their dear "Gompie," as he would become later to Margie's children. They did not mind his silences, his difficulty in communication. They even seemed to accept his convulsive jerking as just something that "Gompie" did.

Life in the little dark apartment was becoming more and more restrictive. Helen was frightened of any disease that attacked the lungs, such as pneumonia, conscious as she was that her mother had nearly died of tuberculosis. Was there any way, any way at all, that she could get a little house—could buy it? When the idea first crossed her mind, she dismissed it. But it kept recurring. Finally she began to pray about it.

"Lord, I don't want to run ahead of You and be presumptuous," she said, "but oh, how I long for my own little home, for a place I can call my own. If there's any way, any way at all, will You show me?"

On the daily level she noticed with a sinking heart that Stan was now deteriorating more rapidly. His originality was pretty well gone. He never made any suggestions. He never said, "Let's do this" or "Let's do that." All the suggestions and planning had to come from Helen. If she said, "Let's go for a ride," he answered meekly, "All right, Mommy."

She tried to make life more interesting for him. She decided that meals should be high points, with the table set as attractively as possible. It was then that she started a mug collection. Each time they went for a drive, if she saw some unusual mugs that were very inexpensive, she would buy two of them. So for meals, Helen frequently used a different mixture of dishes. She found it fun and rewarding. Her love of beauty and art made the pretty table settings vastly satisfying.

Now Helen had to replace Stan's "favorite" chair every year because of his constant violent jerking and twitching. He simply jerked the chairs to pieces. This was an expense for which there was no insurance reimbursement, no medical reimbursement. Unfortunately, his favorites varied, so that he often half-ruined many chairs at a time. Helen tried to set aside funds for replacements, but she always felt that the necessity arose at difficult times.

It became increasingly difficult for Stan to keep from spilling his food or from dropping tools when he tried to effect small household repairs. Often if he was trying to use a tool, he might break whatever he was working with because of his lack of control and jerking motion. But in desperation he continued to insist that he could do anything he chose.

His gait became much worse. During this period it was becoming hard for him to accomplish anything successfully. Helen had bought a small tank of tropical fish to entertain him. He loved them and spent hours watching them dart from place to place among the greenery. At first he had taken the responsibility of changing the water in the tank, though it consumed hours before he was through. As his coordination decreased, Helen found that almost the entire apartment was flooded with water by the time he finished. Another task that she must take over! Finally it was too much for her to do, in addition to all the other work that fell to her lot, and the fish had to be given away, though she knew he would miss them, and it caused her pain.

Now he did not read at all, and something had to be acquired for his entertainment. He could not, she felt, be left in the evenings to sit and twitch convulsively, staring into space. The logical answer—according to friends and family—was a television set.

"But I have never had one and have never had any desire for one," Helen replied. Then she thought about it. Was she being selfish? Should she deprive poor Stan, with his dying mind, of what little pleasure he might derive from watching television? Her heart of love told her that she could not. By careful budgeting, she was able to buy a television set for him.

Almost from the first she wondered how both she and the television set could occupy the same small apartment. Stan would stay up until very, very late, night after night, watching. When he stumbled to bed, knocking into the furniture, he awakened Helen. She could not get back to sleep. Her work at the office was suffering. Stan was still going to his janitorial work each morning, but when he returned in the early afternoon, he slept the hours away to be ready for his night's viewing.

"Stan dearest," she told him one day, as gently as she could, "I think I will have to sleep in the other room. My rest is so disturbed when you come to bed so late."

He gazed at her, full of resentment. "You just don't love me or you wouldn't want to move out of our bedroom!" he exclaimed. "You say you love me, but you really don't."

Bitterly he turned away. She could not reach him. As far as he was concerned, she had rejected him.

Another aspect of the problem was one she did not want to mention to him, since he could do nothing about it. In his sleep, his convulsive jerks were so violent that often he kicked her so hard the pain kept her awake for hours. They had resumed sleeping in a double bed. Poor, poor Stan. How could this horror have come to him? How could it have come to her? Was there never to be release, never a lighthearted moment?

To compensate for what he saw as rejection, Helen began cooking more enthusiastically than she had done in the past. Twice a week she used a new recipe that she had never used before. She tried to vary his diet to make his food interesting as well as nutritious. When she would ask him whether he liked a new dish, he would reply, "Oh, yes, Mommy." Did he really like it? She did not know.

Though he was becoming less a part of the world around him and more absorbed in his half-world of shadows and television, Stan still insisted on keeping the tiny apartment clean. He wouldn't let Helen touch any cleaning. Even the windows sparkled. He still had not lost his love for cleanliness. That would go later.

On Sundays he was always restless, prowling, twitching, jerking. He wanted something to do. He wanted to "go somewhere." Under different circumstances Helen might have taken him to visit friends, but since invitations were no longer extended to them, she shrank from imposing on anyone else. Very well, they would go for "a ride." And so it became an established routine. Every Sunday, as soon as breakfast was over and other small chores done, Stan would turn to her expectantly. "Where are we going today, Mommy?" he would inquire, showing almost the only enthusiasm he ever displayed.

During those years, each containing more than 50 Sundays, Helen felt that she became such an authority on the topography of southern California that she could have gotten a job as a tour guide. She studied maps and brochures and advertisements. During these long hours of driving, Stan never volunteered a remark. He simply sat. If Helen spoke to him, he always answered courteously. But he was somewhere on his own planet.

A new blow came. Helen received a letter one day from her car insurance company, stating that because of Stan's condition, they were canceling the insurance on both her car and Margie's. She knew that if one company canceled out, it would be impossible to reinsure with another company. Her heart beat fast and heavily. If she couldn't drive, she couldn't get to her job; they would be ruined. She knew that only one thing would solve the crisis. She prayed earnestly, then approached Stan.

"Dearest," she said softly, "unless you turn in your driver's license, we won't be able to get any more car insurance. And that will mean I can't drive and Margie can't—and what will we do?"

"I won't give up my license!" he declared heatedly.

And there the matter stood for one day, then two days, then three. Stressful as her life had been for so long, Helen could not remember a more stressful time than this. It seemed to her that every waking moment of every day was one long suspense. Only prayer brought any relief. "You have never forsaken me, dear Lord" was her prayer. "Please work a miracle on Stan's heart."

The Lord gave Helen her miracle. Stan reversed his stand. "I will give up my license for you," he told her. She was stricken to the heart as she realized what a blow this was to his self-esteem, to the remnants of his manhood.

Later, Helen would wonder how the insurance company had known of Stan's condition and would conclude that a "friend" had alerted them. Even when she had the signed slip from the Motor Vehicle Department stating that Stan had surrendered his license, it still took a letter from the union office treasurer to get some insurance for her—this time through the General Conference, which had been briefed by her old friend Elder Blacker as to her crisis.

Dealing with Stan was always like dealing with a willful, stubborn, irresponsible child, yet she knew he was not to blame. His faculties were so impaired, his judgment so distorted, that he could not conceptualize life as it was.

Almost unconsciously Helen, on the Sunday drives, began noticing "For Sale" signs. Idly she would think to herself, "I wonder how much that house is selling for?" "I wonder what is the price of that little piece of land?" But she didn't really organize her thoughts until one day it struck her that she had a golden opportunity now to find another little piece of property! Surely no real-estate agent could cover the territory more thoroughly than she was covering it. If by some miracle she could get another piece of land in a way similar to the one she had gotten near Sonora, she could squeeze out another monthly payment, somehow, some way.

Almost as though the Lord had arranged it, one sunny Sunday she and Stan were riding through a beautiful little valley in the vicinity of Lancaster and Palmdale.

"Daddy, it's like being in a teacup," she smiled at Stan. "It's so green and the background mountains are so beautiful."

Then, almost in the same breath, she exclaimed, "Why don't we buy a lot in here if we can?"

Stan's eyes focused on her. "Yes, that would be nice," he agreed passively.

But even Stan's passivity couldn't dampen Helen's new-found enthusiasm. Before she could lose her courage, she stopped at the first real-estate office, which was open. When she explained to the realtor what she was hoping for, the latter told her (in the classic way realtors have), "Why, I know just the place for you!"

It was.

The lot had oak trees, beautiful manzanita, water, and a perfect building site for a house. In this particular area of California, water was especially important. So Helen used the remaining $200 of her savings as a down payment and made arrangements for small monthly payments. For the first time since Stan had left home and then returned she began to feel a little sense of security, a little lessening of her concern for the future. "How can two little pieces of land make such a difference?" she asked herself.

When Helen had taken her father back to Reno, when she had realized that she could not care for both him and Stan in the small apartment, she had assumed he would return to his little home where he and her mother had lived for all their married life. She had said to him, "Dad, you took care of Mother for years, when she was young and had tuberculosis and then in the last years of her life when she was feeble. You've done the cooking. You have a nice little home and you're comfortable. You know nearly everyone in Reno, or so it seems to me. I know it will never be the same without Mother, but I think you can have some moments of happiness."

But it hadn't worked out that way. He had been far more emotionally dependent on his wife than any of the children had realized. In addition, he developed a morbid feeling of guilt because he was driving when the accident occurred. "I killed Mother," he would weep, over and over. He refused to cook for himself, to care for his person as he should; finally Harry, in Reno, made arrangements for him to live in an old people's home. Still he cried all the time, and begged to be taken to his wife's grave every day.

When Helen received the telephone call telling of his death, she did not realize that the circumstances surrounding it would bring her more sorrow, more grief. As the story unfolded, her conscience again smote her. Should she have kept him with her? Should she have tried to be the answer to more problems, in spite of the advice of the psychiatrist?

Her father had gotten up very early one morning, gone to those in charge, and begged for his medication. They replied, "But the medication is due at breakfast. You must wait until then." Other patients, listening, reported that the nurses had been very unkind, very impatient.

When breakfast time came, his condition had deteriorated to the point that he could not walk to the dining room. The nurse on duty was adamant.

"We will not bring your breakfast to the room; you're perfectly able to get up and walk, and if you think you're going to get away with this kind of thing, you're wrong!" she shouted at him.

Overhearing these words, two tiny, frail, elderly ladies, friends of Ben Sanford, went into the room when the nurse had gone.

"Ben," they begged, leaning over his bed, "let us help you to the dining room. We'll walk on either side of you."

He looked up at them, his eyes unfocused, obviously not himself. But he summoned his last shred of strength, sat up, and finally was on his feet. The three of them approached the dining room in this fashion, only to be greeted at the doors by shouts and jeers.

"Ben Sanford! You big old man—how can you let two little ladies help you into the dining room!" were words that cut into his heart.

By ten o'clock that morning he was in a coma. The last words he ever heard were the cruel jibes. He who had been kind to others, who had given so many needy people help, in his extremity was given only scorn.

Helen's sobs, as she finally learned the entire story, racked her body. The pent-up tears that she held back, day after day, came in a flood. It seemed to her she could not bear this additional sadness, could not ever make peace with such cruelty. And as the years passed, her grief on that account did not really lessen. Thoughts of her father's death always brought tears.

The two apartments in the little house were rented. She and her two brothers were the heirs, and the small check Helen now received each month was a significant help. When later her niece bought the house and she received a few thousand dollars in cash, she promptly put the money in the bank. How much better she felt, with that small "cushion."

June 28, 1968. This was a day Helen had dreaded, though she had not known what the exact date would be. She had known only that the time would come when Stan could no longer work, when he could no longer carry on his janitorial duties. The incident that brought the decision seemed small at first—severe warts on the bottoms of both his feet. He couldn't walk without limping. When a young doctor removed them, his flesh seemed unable to heal. He was in agony, still hobbling to his job each day, creeping along behind his mops and brooms and vacuum cleaner. Helen couldn't bear to see him struggle any longer.

"Stan dear," she said to him, "you don't have to suffer like this. The time has come when I think you should quit work. You will have the sustentation benefits that you accumulated in the ministry and as an employee at the hospital, and Social Security disability payments. With what I make, we will manage."

She had expected that he would protest, might even refuse. But he did not. He seemed to realize that he was at the end of another phase of his life. But his last day as an Adventist worker was a sad one for Helen. Where were all the glowing plans of her youth? Where had it all gone, the glory and the dreams?

"Well, at least one of my dreams came true," Helen told herself, wiping away secret tears. "When I was a young girl I used to think it would be marvelous to be secretary to a conference president or a union president, and now I'm secretary to the president of the Pacific Union!" Helen had assumed this position some time previously.

As the last day of Stan's employment had approached, Helen had again reviewed all their finances. She added up the funds they would have received in educational benefits if Stan's illness had been diagnosed and he had not felt he had to run away. She sat and thought of the terrible financial losses they had suffered. She thought of the future, in which she would need so much money to provide proper care for him. And eventually, could she provide for herself? She decided to make a last appeal for a reconsideration of her case, based on the fact that Stan was incurably ill, that he had been incurably ill when he left, and that the statements of his doctors were proof of this.

With much prayer and careful thought, she composed a letter explaining in detail what she had lost and what she hoped for. She expressed the longing of her heart for less insecurity, for some ray of hope. She outlined what she had been told to expect in the way of future expenses for Stan. With yet another prayer, she sealed the envelope and sent it on its way.

The letter was never answered. For weeks Helen's heart beat expectantly each day when the mail came across her office desk or when she picked up the mail at home. Then through the office "grapevine" she heard it had been decided that her letter would simply be filed.

The blow was staggering. If only she had been told kindly and sympathetically that nothing could be done for her. If only! As she looked around her, privy as she was to all the financial matters of the office, and saw special appropriations being given to this one and to that one and saw the lavish travel budgets and other allowances, she had to struggle with a brief period of bitterness. Then prayer again was her answer. After a session on her knees, she arose with a new attitude.

"Well, Lord, here we are again, just the two of us," she told God. "I think the committee would be blessed if they would reconsider my request, but since they won't I claim Your promise that You have a thousand ways to provide for me."

A goal of Helen's became the education of executives in the church to the need of circumventing policy on certain occasions, when the facts of a case were not clear-cut. She hoped to prevent another person's being hurt as she had been.

Still longing for a further outlet in the dark apartment and still missing social life, Helen implemented her lifelong dream when she enrolled in a bona fide art class. She discovered that Glendale City College offered special adult-education courses, with an art class meeting in an elementary school only about a mile away. She heard about this opportunity a bit late, and when she tried to enroll she found that all the classes were filled—except a class in portrait painting.

"I have never had a class in art since junior high," she told the instructor.

"Well, why not see what you can do with it?" was the reply.

Helen entered the world of live models and posing and charcoal drawings and found to her chagrin that she couldn't even get the heads of her people to seem round! But she stuck with it, and at the end of the semester she could see a great deal of improvement in her work.

"Who knows? Maybe I can make some money someday with my art," she chattered to Stan, who did not reply. Perhaps he did not really hear.

Her appetite having been whetted by the two small lots she was buying, Helen began to think in terms of someday building a house out in Green Valley. When she found that the lot adjoining hers was for sale, she bought it also, with almost no down payment and small monthly payments. But she realized that it was too far from her work.

Her prayers began to have the word *house* in them over and over. "Lord, You know how much better it would be for us if we had a house," she prayed. "Is it presumptuous of me to think of such a thing?"

Almost as though someone had answered aloud, the words came into her mind, "If you find something for under $20,000."

Almost automatically she spoke aloud. "But no one in the *world* could buy a house here in southern California for less than $20,000!"

Again the conviction, stronger than ever. "Look for a house under $20,000."

But even if she—by a miracle no less dramatic than the feeding of the five thousand—should find such a house, where would she get a down payment? She wondered why this vital item had escaped her notice until now. What was the matter with her? Was her mind also going?

Suddenly, like a flash of lightning, she had the answer. The second mortgage on the house in Oakland! Stan had left her that when he took everything else. It was to have been paid off long ere now in a lump sum, but it hadn't been. Could she manage to get the lump sum? If so, perhaps it would be enough for a down payment on the modest place she must find.

She did get the lump sum, with the help of a friendly lawyer. Electrified, she started looking in earnest, on every lunch hour and early evening. But the houses she found for her price were so dirty, so unkempt, so totally awful in every way, that she almost began to believe that she had imagined the Lord's leading. On the day that she saw one of the most depressing houses on her lunch hour, she plodded back to the office, her spirits drooping. Her friend from whom she had bought the five acres was waiting for her.

"Helen," she exclaimed excitedly, "I saw *your* house today. You must go to see it tonight. I think we would buy it for ourselves, but the bedroom's too small for a king-size bed. But somehow the house just looks like you, Helen. I tell you—it's your house!"

The afternoon hours at the typewriter dragged. When five o'clock came, Helen, with a fast-beating heart, drove to La Crescenta, a small suburb in the hills above Glendale. "Oh, please, Lord, please let this be my house," she begged silently.

As though coming home from a long journey, Helen recognized the house. It was "hers." True, there were enormous amounts of work to be done. But the overall charm was so great that Helen drank it in. The house had been built about thirty years ago up in the oaks as a weekend retreat, probably by a wealthy homeowner in the elite suburb of Beverly Hills. There was a large living room, a large fireplace, box windows. From the living room one stepped up into a little dining room with two enchanting doors that opened into a study, with built-in bookshelves to the ceiling. The kitchen was paneled with wood. At the back of the house was another room that had obviously been added after the original construction, paneled in knotty pine, with an open-beam ceiling. Though the house contained only about a thousand square feet, to Helen it was a mansion.

She rushed home to get Stan. As she took him through, she kept saying, "Isn't it lovely, Stan? Wouldn't you like to live here?"

He mumbled that he didn't see why they had to leave the apartment. Actually, this had been a problem. Stan had exhibited a good deal of resentment over Helen's conviction that they needed to purchase a small home. It seemed utterly impossible for her to get through to him regarding their precarious financial situation. And she would not, could not, bring up the subject of his future institutionalization. That would be too cruel.

"Well, I like it, and I'm going to make an offer," she told him.

The asking price was $22,500—above Helen's prayer figure. She made an offer of $19,000. The owners countered with $19,500.

"It's a deal!" Helen announced.

She was not to know that in addition to all the repair and redecorating work, the roof would leak the next winter and she would have to figure out financing for a new roof! Once in the house, Stan roused himself from his lethargy and gave Helen a great deal of help. When the house began to take on the look Helen loved (polished and shining), she started work on the yard, already beautiful with a clump of oaks, ferns, and camellias. In front was a little split-rail fence. After the first few months, when Helen would stand outside and look around her, she would feel tears of gladness in her eyes. At one time she had thought she would never have another home. But now she did. God was good. The devil did not fully prevail.

Moreover, after she was well settled into the house in La Crescenta, she found a buyer for the lots in Green Valley. To her joy, she cleared enough to pay off her second mortgage, so that she owed only $15,000 on her home. Turning her bankbook over to God had been the best fiscal decision of her life, she often said to herself.

In addition to her little home, Helen had Margie's first baby—little Becky—to bring her joy. Loma Linda was close enough for frequent visiting. Stan loved the baby. In spite of his emotional instability, his outbursts, his convulsive jerking, around the baby he seemed more relaxed. It was a real deprivation when Margie and her husband accepted a position in the Midwest, so far from California.

Helen tried to monitor Stan's activities as closely as she could, though if they were to continue living, she must spend her days in her office. He adopted the habit of walking to a small nearby café for lunch. Since he obviously enjoyed this so much and since the patrons of the café seemed to accept him, Helen did not mind the extra expense. Sometimes in the afternoons he would go to the nearby public library, often checking out books, particularly on art and history.

His muscular coordination now was totally unreliable. When Helen, away on a short errand one Sunday, returned home and found him up on a high ladder, pruning trees, the ladder propped very precariously, her heart was in her mouth. And with good reason, for in a few short moments the ladder slipped and Stan fell, landing heavily on his shoulder. He was instantly in severe pain. Helen rushed him to Glendale Adventist Hospital. Diagnosis: broken shoulder blade. Treatment: a month in the hospital.

Now a new facet of Stan's tragedy became clear. He was totally incapable of lying still. In the hospital bed his arms and legs jerked and twitched ceaselessly, night and day.

"He'll be in agony with bedsores!" gasped the head nurse of Stan's floor after only twenty-four hours. "We have to do something, think up something."

The "something" turned out to be pillows pinned all over his bed—pinned to his pajamas, whenever possible. "At least the pillows will keep the friction from being so great during his constant moving," the nurses agreed.

But the month he spent in the hospital was terrible for him, terrible for those who cared for him. At times he seemed eager to cooperate. At other times he seemed not to care. Mixed with her concern for him, Helen felt almost a sense of relief. Each night when she went home he was not sitting in his chair, twitching, twitching, jerking, watching TV or simply staring into space. He was well taken care of. For the first time since he had returned and his illness had been diagnosed she felt that she could relax. She could take long, leisurely baths. She couldn't have enjoyed any of these privileges if she had felt that he was being neglected or if she had felt that she had arbitrarily placed him in the care of others. Circumstances had given her a month's reprieve.

After his shoulder healed—and his doctor told Helen that probably no other bone in Stan's body could have healed, because of his constant motion—he returned to his "routine," his café lunches, his TV watching, his silence, punctuated by outbursts that were becoming irrational at times. From time to time he seemed to be confused as to who Helen was. Was she his mother? Was she his wife?

Then Margie's new baby arrived in the Midwest; she needed Helen, who had arranged to take her vacation to care for Margie and the baby. Helen had wondered what she would do with Stan. He solved the problem by insisting that he wanted to go along, so somehow, someway Helen managed the money for the two plane tickets.

He was ecstatic at being with Margie, his dearest darling, and little Becky and newborn Jamie. He seemed to be having the best time he had had in years. He showed so many flashes of the old endearing Stan that Helen's heart was soft with love and remembrance.

Then suddenly, with no warning, he suffered one of his lightning changes of mood. "We've been here long enough," he announced to Helen. "We're going home right away."

It was never wise to cross him when he was in one of those moods. But Margie needed her mother. Helen still had a week of her vacation. In a rare show of spunk, she said to Stan, "All right, you can go home if you want to, but I'm staying. I'll take you to the airport—but what will you do when you reach Los Angeles?"

This spirited response seemed to calm him. He said nothing further about leaving. But as he took little Becky walking, Margie pointed out to Helen that his movements were the most violent she had seen. She also sadly noted that he could not bear for anyone to cross him, to disagree with him.

"Mother," Margie said, "I think you'd better get ready for the fact that very soon Daddy will be more than you can handle."

Though Helen knew that the words were true, she cringed inwardly. For so long she had dreaded what was to come, and now, apparently, it was soon to be a reality.

Just about the time that Helen had gotten the house to look as pretty as she'd hoped and arranged all her few keepsakes on shelves, including the lovely china she'd painted in her class, the earthquake of February 21, 1971, took place. When the earth began to shake and move violently during the early morning, Helen's first confused thoughts were of Stan. He fell so often; it seemed that she was always running to help him. Now she wondered what would become of him. He would panic. Around her she could hear constant crashings as her dishes slid from the shelves, the keepsakes fell from their racks, and other loose objects went in all directions. With the speed and concentration one acquires in moments of crisis, Helen dashed through the broken glass and china of the kitchen, not even considering that she might cut herself badly. (Later she found that miraculously she had only one cut.) She reached Stan, put her arms around him, and they sat together on the side of the bed. Around them the crashing, crashing, crashing continued.

When the terrifying heaving and swaying of the earth stopped, they made their way outside. Later they would wonder why they hadn't stayed inside where perhaps it was safer, but they, along with all their neighbors, seemed to have an uncontrollable urge to seek the freedom of the outdoors, as though here they might find accustomed stability. The drugstore near them met their eye—a shambles. A house only one block away was obviously so badly damaged that later it was taken down—a beautiful stone house, just purchased, whose new owners had lovingly spent uncalculated time and money fixing it up.

As they stood in the street in their nightwear, shivering, along with their neighbors, Helen suddenly noticed a curl of smoke spiraling upward from a shed across the street from their house.

"The shed is on fire!" she shouted. "I must phone for the fire department!"

"All the phones are out of order," the neighbors told her.

"But maybe mine isn't," was Helen's swift reply as she raced into the house. With a fast-beating heart, she picked up the phone, held it to her ear—and heard one of the sweetest sounds of her life—the familiar dial tone. Later she would learn that hers was indeed the only house in that area whose phone still worked. Miraculously, the fire-department trucks were not tied up yet with other fires; their swift appearance and efficient service curtailed what would have been a major tragedy if the large oak trees had caught fire.

Soon it was time for Helen to go to her office.

"I'll clean up the mess while you are at work," Stan mumbled to Helen as she gave him his breakfast.

"Oh, you don't need to do that. I've already swept the china and glass out of the kitchen, and when I get home we'll work together," she told him.

He said nothing. She realized, with a sinking heart, that he was in one of his more stubborn moods and was in a state of shock. What would he do with their things? His judgment was so uncertain. But, tired and sleepless as she was, she didn't feel capable of facing a screaming confrontation.

Her heart in her mouth, she opened the front door in the late afternoon. Stan was sitting in front of the television. The house looked orderly. She thanked him profusely for his work. Only later, when she began looking for prized possessions, did she discover he had thrown things out wildly, including precious books that could never be replaced.

Helen's chief regret was for the few pieces of Haviland china she had inherited from her mother. They had belonged to her paternal grandmother, deceased before her mother and father married. "These lovely dishes will be yours, Helen," her mother had told her many times.

It hadn't worked out that way, though. At her mother's death, Helen was so burdened with the care of Stan that she hadn't been able to stay in Reno and go through the cupboards. Since everyone in the family had for years referred to the china as "Helen's Haviland," she had assumed that arrangements would be made to send it. Alas, only recently had a few dishes gotten into her possession. And now Stan had thrown the pieces of the broken ones away. Could some have been repaired? She would never know. There were still a few, very few, dishes remaining!

All Stan's life he had yearned to know more about his mother's family. He seemed to feel rootless. Though he appreciated the love and care of his foster parents and respected and loved them in return, something was missing, some vital link with the past. Many times he had tried, without success, to locate the graves of his maternal grandparents. He had always wondered why, when his mother died, they had not taken him as their own. In the spring of 1971, through the most fortuitous of circumstances, Helen stumbled across clues that led her to Stan's aunts (whom he had never seen) and finally to the cemetery where his mother's parents were buried. When they drove into the cemetery and parked, Stan made his wishes clear.

"I want to go by myself to find the graves," he told Helen. Through misted eyes, she agreed. She watched him stumbling and staggering back and forth among the graves, her heart too full for tears. When finally he found his grandfather's grave, he stood beside it for a long time. Helen felt that emotional healing took place when the wonderings of his life were answered. He knew for the first time that his grandfather had died before he was born.

Finally he staggered back, got into the car, and sat silently. Helen started the motor. Never again did he refer to the incident.

Stan's moods sank deeper and deeper. He sat for hours, saying nothing. At times he responded to Helen's conversation; at other times he did not. Then he began to make threats on his life.

"I'd be better off dead, and you'd be better off if I were dead," he muttered to Helen one night.

An icy finger touched her heart.

"No, no, Stan!" she cried. "Don't say that—please don't even think it. I love you, and Jacquee and her children love you, and so do Margie and her children . . ."

The mention of the grandchildren seemed to reach him. "Gompie" was dear to them; they accepted him. Perhaps he found his only solace in their uncritical company, his only ease in their uncomplicated love.

Helen hoped that he had forgotten his threats. He hadn't. A few days later he calmly announced, "I've taken enough sleeping pills to kill me, and that's the way I want it."

Terrified, Helen rushed for his pill bottle. She had long learned that his remarks were not always to be taken at face value. When she saw that the level of pills had not gone down appreciably, she was relieved. Stan slept for a long time during the afternoon, but otherwise suffered no ill effects.

This was a scene that was repeated several times, but Helen's nerves were always taut. She never knew just what she would find when she came home from work. The disease with all its implications was closing in on both of them. Now she hid his medications or locked them in a secure place, giving him only his daily amounts.

He had become hostile to her, once his adored "Snooksie." He seemed to regard her a great deal of the time as his enemy, as one who plotted against him. Though she had been warned that this development was inevitable, Helen wept bitter tears. Where, where was her young and handsome Stan, the boy who had worked his hands to actual rawness to pay for their second baby? Where had it all gone?

Now it was the early spring of 1971. It was more evident to Helen every day that she must make decisions about Stan's future and that she would also have to be in a position to do what must be done for him. Until now, she had permitted him to sign checks, to cosign papers for the house, the car, and other legal matters. But now he was slipping downhill so fast, his mind so clouded, that the future was ominous.

Taking her courage in her hands, Helen said to him one evening, "Stan, my dearest, will you let me file a power of attorney so that we can both know that in the future I can be sure you have proper care and everything is done that should be done?"

Fearfully she waited for his answer. She still did not know how much he understood, or whether at any given time she was talking to the sane Stan, or to the dreadful impostor who lived in his body.

Finally he answered. One word. "Yes."

As his disease progressed, she was always grateful that she had taken this precaution in time.

One bright spot on Stan's darkening horizon was Jacquee's unflagging love and attention. Moreover, her second husband was the soul of kindness, the soul of consideration. At least every three months the little family came to visit. Howard's gentle teasing could bring appreciative smiles to Stan's face in a way that nothing else could. Sometimes Helen would see him gazing at his firstborn, his face so open and vulnerable, so full of love, that she would turn away with a lump in her throat.

One day that spring as she took him for a drive out near the town of Camarillo, he turned to her and, with no preface, made a statement that chilled her to the marrow.

"I want you to commit me to the State hospital here in Camarillo," he told her.

"But, Stan!" she gasped.

"No, that's what I want you to do," he insisted stubbornly, his voice rising in the whining inflection that was a danger signal. Hastily she agreed that she would investigate the possibility.

"I want you to talk to them right now," he insisted. There was nothing to do but drive to the hospital.

When Helen explained Stan's situation to the interviewer, she was told that the matter couldn't be handled that way. "Mr. Jefferson will have to go to the University of Southern California Hospital, turn himself in there (or you turn him in), and they will commit him. Eventually he will end up here."

She had thought Stan might have changed his mind, but he had not. "Take me to USC," he mumbled, twitching and convulsing.

At the USC Hospital he signed himself in—scribbled

himself in, actually, since his handwriting had long ago become illegible—and walked away from Helen without a backward glance, following a nurse who had taken him in charge.

Helen went home to the empty house, an emptiness different from any other she had experienced. She had gone through Stan's leaving home, but then there had been Margie. Now she was all alone. In spite of the constant care and constant problem Stan presented, he was a living presence. In spite of his frequent hostility to her, he was her husband. He was the center of her life in every way. She stood in the living room of the little home that they had both worked so hard on, and sobbed.

Then she sank to her knees. "Dear Father," she prayed, "if this isn't the time for Stan to go into an institution, please make that clear. I don't want to send him away from his home one moment sooner than he must go. Please overrule in every way so that only the right things will be done. Please be near my poor, tortured Stan in that strange hospital."

She spent a restless, sleepless night and could hardly wait for the end of her workday so that she could drive to the hospital, alone, as always, it seemed. When she found that Stan had been placed in a ward with twelve other men, some of them uncouth, repulsive, and profane, her heart sank.

"Stan, I don't want you to stay here," she told him.

He seemed lucid. "But they're going to give me lots of tests, and I want to see what the tests reveal," he told her.

When, at the end of the week, the tests confirmed the diagnosis—yet again—of Huntington's chorea, the doctors at the USC Hospital signed papers to commit Stan to Camarillo State Hospital.

"I don't see how I can take him there!" Helen told them.

"But, Mrs. Jefferson, soon you will have no choice," they told her. "Soon he will be uncontrollable."

But when she took Stan to the car, both of them cried bitterly. With his remaining sensibilities, he didn't want to leave her. He seemed loving, gentle. He dreaded the end of his life, so to speak, the end of all his freedom, all his miniscule pleasures. Finally Helen dried her eyes.

"Come on, darling, we're going home," she announced, and like a weary child, he put his head back against the seat of the car and dozed.

But taking him home was a mistake. The summer heat was more than he could bear. The nerves on the outside of his body, which were as raw as tortured flesh, were matched by the nerves inside his body in the same condition. He was literally a body in hell. Helen took some of her slender savings to buy an air conditioner for his bedroom, but the noise rubbed on his sensibilities so that he could not endure it.

In addition to the torture of the air conditioner, he complained constantly about his stomach. "My stomach, my stomach," he would mutter, rolling on his bed, clutching his abdomen, his face contorted. He refused nearly all food. He began to waste away alarmingly.

Again there was a trip to the doctor (how many had she made with him during these years?) and the attempt to diagnose his problem while he, incoherent, could not explain the nature of either his pain or the foods he was convinced bothered him most. Then there was the stop at the drugstore for the filling of his prescriptions (how many times had she done this?). The medicine cabinet by now would not have held all his medicines, though in many cases he had taken only one or two pills or several spoonfuls and declared the prescription worthless.

Helen, though, had continued to keep all his former medications hidden as his determination to kill himself seemed to harden. Now he had a new prescription. She had not thought to ask the doctor what effect a massive overdose might have, not relating the thought of stomach medication to suicide. When, on July 29, she came home at noon to check on him and found him unconscious on his bed, she was anguished. She tried to rouse him, shouting his name. No response. She rubbed his arms, cold as death. No response.

Flying to the phone, she called the rescue squad, who arrived with sirens screaming, a police car accompanying them. Neighbors came out into their yards and watched the paramedics bring Stan out on a stretcher and start for the hospital, but not until after the police officer and the medics had tried as hard as possible to rouse him.

After first aid had been given to him at the hospital and Helen had filled out what seemed to her almost miles of official-looking forms, she was allowed to see him.

Weak as he was, his limbs twitching and jerking, his face in convulsive spasms, he still managed a little smile, which broke her heart.

"I wonder why I took all those pills, Mommy," he whispered.

Helen could not forgive herself for having overlooked this possibility. Yet, with one corner of her mind, she wondered whether he would not have been better off had he succeeded. He was doomed to the most intense suffering, the most degrading of lives. Was it surprising that he wanted to end it? Should not a human being be allowed to exit this life with dignity?

But she sternly repressed those thoughts. God is the life-giver. He is the one who numbers our days, she told herself. In her seasons of prayer, which were her strength and solace, she begged the Lord to give Stan the fortitude that he must have. "Please don't let him suffer so much," she prayed, "and help him not to be so keenly aware of what's happening to him. And give me patience, Lord, and an extra measure of love."

CHAPTER 15
Stan's Worsening Condition

NOW began a period of intense trial, as Stan's condition worsened daily. Helen had to take care of the endless family business, the filling out of forms, the applying for benefits, the complicated medical claims, the planning, the thinking. Often this had to be done over and beyond Stan's violent objections, his increasing paranoia where she was concerned. He longed for Margie, the loving, understanding daughter he had cherished so tenderly.

"But Margie is in the Midwest, Daddy," Helen told him gently over and over. "I know you want to see her, but she has two little children and she has her husband. Do you want me to take you to visit her?"

He would mumble something, and the matter would rest until he again expressed longing to see her. He brightened at Jacquee's and Howard's regular visits.

As long as Helen's physical strength and well-being continued at a fairly good level, she was able to cope. But now her back, never fully recovered from the fracture of her coccyx bone suffered years before, began to pain her so cruelly that she was almost incapacitated. Friends at the office, noticing that she would grimace in pain when she attempted to stand, or walk for any length of time, or bend over, voiced their concern.

"Helen, you simply have to get some medical attention for that back," they would tell her.

"Oh, I think I can wear it out before it wears me out" was her standard reply.

But when she got to the point that she actually groaned in agony each time she sat for any length of time and then attempted to stand, she was at last driven to make an appointment with a doctor.

After examinations, X-rays, and tests, her doctor said, "You will have to have surgery on your back. There is simply no other way."

"But, doctor, there's no one to look after my husband. I don't know how I can manage," Helen cried in frustration, pain, and apprehension.

"He can stay alone for a week," her doctor told her gently. "It's time you thought of yourself a little."

Encouraged by his concern for her welfare, Helen made her arrangements. When she broached the matter to Stan, he was almost unconcerned.

"I will take care of myself. Don't worry about me," he mumbled, then turned away and fastened his attention again on the TV screen.

"I'll cook little casseroles and put them in the refrigerator, and all you will have to do is put them in the oven and you'll have a meal," Helen told him cheerfully, far more cheerfully than she felt. She knew that he couldn't even slice tomatoes, his coordination was now so impaired.

At last preparations were made. His food was cooked and in the refrigerator. The hospital arrangements were made. The surgery was set for the next day. Her office arrangements had been completed. With all this resting on her shoulders, Helen hadn't had the opportunity to become apprehensive about the spinal surgery, which was just as well, she thought to herself.

With her bag packed, she came into the living room. "Daddy," she said to Stan, "let's have prayer together, and then I will drive myself to the hospital."

They knelt and prayed. That is, Helen prayed. Midway through her prayer he began to sob uncontrollably. She put her arms around him.

"Don't worry, Stan. I'll be all right," she comforted him.

"I'm not worried about you!" he burst out. "I just can't

stay here by myself. I can't! I can't!"

Seeing his frantic agitation and lack of control, Helen's heart sank. Now what could she do? She could not send him to Jacquee, in northern California, nor to Margie, in the Midwest. Both had their own problems and their young families. Her brothers could not take him, because of family circumstances.

She grabbed the phone book, turned to the heading "Convalescent Hospitals," and began going down the list, trying to find the ones nearest Glendale. As she dialed, her thoughts were in a turmoil. How would she pay for his care in one of those hospitals? Would her insurance cover most of it? Did any of them take patients on a short-stay basis? How could it be worked out?

At place after place, she received a negative answer. No, we don't make that sort of arrangement. No, sorry. No, try us again sometime. No. Just when she was about to surrender to total discouragement and cancel her surgery, she heard the word Yes. And then there was the rushing around, the packing of his necessities, the driving him to the convalescent hospital, the filling out of forms (how many had she filled out during this year?), and then, breathless and perspiring, she turned her car toward Glendale Adventist Hospital. By four in the afternoon she checked herself in (more forms to fill out) and settled into a hospital bed with a long sigh of relief. Even the stream of hospital people through her room, lab technicians, interns, nurses, dietitians, et cetera, did not seem worrisome. After all, she was relaxed. Stan was being taken care of. For these precious hours she had surrendered her burden.

When, sometime the next day, she awoke from her surgery, she wondered, as so many surgical patients often wonder, why she had consented to the operation. Her lower back was on fire. She couldn't lie on either hip. She couldn't lie flat on her back. She couldn't lie on her stomach. The first three days were a blur of pain, nausea, injections, and interludes of unconsciousness. Then slowly she began to return to the real world, only to find herself worrying incessantly about the high price of the convalescent hospital for Stan, knowing that there was no insurance that would cover the charges. For that matter, her own expenses would not be fully covered.

When, after constant pleading on Helen's part, her doctor consented for her to leave the hospital, she found that she couldn't drive her car home, for the rather simple reason that she couldn't sit down. The lower part of her spine had been so bruised by the surgery that sitting was out of the question.

"Will you drive me home in my car and circle around to the convalescent hospital and get Stan?" she hesitantly asked a friend who had phoned. Helen found it difficult to ask for help, even at this late date and in her extremity of need. Her early home training had never left her.

"Of course I will," her friend replied warmly. Helen half-crouched on one leg during the ride home, which was, to her, excruciatingly painful.

Stan seemed stolid, remote, unaffected by his stay in the hospital and indifferent to his reunion with her. His convulsive twitching and jerking were constant during the day. Only in deep sleep did relief ever come to him. When her friend had left the two of them, her heart heavy with knowledge of Helen's burdens, Helen was almost overwhelmed.

"I'm so much weaker than I thought I would be," she whispered to herself. "How can I take care of Stan? How can I cook for him and control him?"

She lay in her bed and prayed, hour after hour. Stan sat in front of the television set, oblivious to everything else. As the days passed, Helen developed a serious infection in her incision. Stan was too uncoordinated to help her with her medication. She almost despaired.

Margie, though, with her usual perception where her

mother was concerned, realized that things were not good. As a nurse, she knew all too well what kind of surgery Helen had undergone. She phoned. "Mother, John and I are coming to be with you and Daddy for a little while" was the welcome message.

How much better Helen felt! Her one concern was that she couldn't scrub the bathtub as sparkling as she wished it to be. Her back was almost forgotten in the problem of the tub.

"Stan," she said with a flash of inspiration, "here is some money. I want you to go down to the corner store and buy me a new mop."

He was still able to do errands of this kind, from time to time, though had she been in better physical condition, she probably would not have asked him. Surprisingly enough, he returned in short order with just the mop she needed.

Brightly she wrung it out in the sink, and *mopped* the tub, using scouring powder until the tub shone like a mirror!

"Stan," she laughed, "do you think I ought to get some kind of prize for an inventive mind?"

He gazed at her silently, uncomprehending.

Oh, the blessedness of being with Margie! Oh, the joy of having this child of hers, so understanding, so loving, to lean on, for just a little while. Helen began to recover.

"Mother," Margie said to her one day, as they sat alone together, "I think you must resign yourself to putting Daddy into an institution very soon. I know you almost made the decision once before, but I can't tell you how much he has deteriorated since last I saw him. You mustn't wait until you can't handle him—until he goes berserk and hurts himself or you or others."

Helen felt the tears forming in her eyes and the lump in her throat.

"But most of the places are so awful," she whispered. "They smell of urine. The patients are sitting there waiting to die. How can I abandon Daddy to one of them?"

Now Margie's own eyes were full of tears. "I know—I

know. But there's just no other way."

To her father, Margie was as loving and gentle as always. He found his keenest joy in the two little children, the little girl and boy. They hugged "Gompie" and tagged after him and seemed to take it as a matter of course that his arms and legs were always jerking and twitching and his head snapping back and forth and his face contorting.

With the children and Margie and John, Stan seemed more in control of his emotions. He did not make threats upon his life. He did not shout and go into tantrums.

But their visit came to an end. Helen went back to the office, barely able to sit at her desk. She had been away from work for six weeks, and she must earn money if Stan and she were to continue living.

The days went by. They turned into weeks. Now Stan's mind seemed dark, hopeless, confused. Helen could not get him out of bed in the mornings. He was no longer able to bathe himself or shave. He was becoming more and more a stranger to her. Her own dear Stan was gone forever, prey to a cruel invader.

When, one day, he cried for hours and would not listen to any reason, any cajolings, she knew that Margie had been right. The time had come. The previous day she had prayed, in her extremity, "Lord, if the time has come for Stan now to be in the care of others, please make it clear to me. I don't want to make a mistake." And the Lord had made it clear.

Earlier Stan had expressed a desire to be put into an institution where he could be given a vegetarian diet, though he had wavered between vegetarianism and meat-eating for years, depending upon his stomach problems.

"I'm going to make arrangements with Simi Valley," Helen told him, and was intensely relieved when the administrator agreed that they would take Stan. What a nice place it was! Helen went through the familiar but never-simple process of filling out forms, forms, forms. Then there were consultations when she had to show all Stan's previous medical records, the latter now a large and bulky envelope.

"If only one doctor could carry through on his case," she often said to herself.

Throughout Stan's long and expensive illness, Helen had been first surprised, then wounded, by the large bills presented to her by nearly every doctor who treated him, no matter how briefly or how superficially. She had known many of these doctors socially; some were friends of Margie's from her Loma Linda training days. She had hoped for some consideration; she had hoped that they would understand her lack of funds and lack of full medical assistance from the church. Too proud to mention her situation, she juggled her meager resources and met every bill on time.

"It isn't that I think doctors aren't worthy of their hire," she told a friend when a particularly large bill came in, panicking her for the moment. "It's just that I wish they could see what a burden it is for someone in my situation."

One bright spot during the years was a hospital in Duarte named "City of Hope." For Helen, it was true to its name. This hospital, on finding out the situation, never charged for Stan's care as an outpatient; the doctors on the staff gave their services as a humanitarian gesture. If only she could have taken him there at all times, she thought, but the distance was sometimes a problem and whatever doctor treated him at a given time had his own favorite medical facilities. The Duarte hospital, a research center for rare and terminal diseases, especially neurological and cancerous, was nondenominational, but to Helen it was truly Christian.

After she had Stan settled in his room at Simi, Helen again experienced the heavy sadness of leaving him. He looked so pitiful. Would he be treated with sympathy and consideration? Would those caring for him realize that he was not responsible for his conduct, which at times bordered on the subhuman?

When she made the arrangements for him to be admitted, with all the complicated paper work, Helen had made it clear that Stan could not, no matter how rational he might appear at times, ever be allowed to have his medications in his possession. His attempts on his life had convinced her that such an impulse might strike him at any time.

During his first hospitalizations Helen had been told that she must buy his medications herself and bring them to the hospital. This meant that once a month she made a trip to the pharmacy, had the prescriptions filled, took them to his hospital, searched out the person in charge of Stan's ward, and made sure that the medications were given to him or her.

She went through the long explanation at Simi; she would go through it at every subsequent facility where he was a patient. Then she would lose sleep wondering whether the persons in charge had given him his medicine, which he so badly needed to keep him controllable.

As she drove the long distance from Simi Valley to Glendale on the crowded freeways, Helen's heart was too heavy for tears. The wheels seemed to repeat over and over the refrain "You've deserted him; you've deserted him; you've deserted him," until she almost cried aloud in her torment. A quick petition heavenward brought blessed relief. It was as though a voice spoke saying, "But Helen, you must work to pay his bills. You can no longer keep him at home and do this. You have loved and cared for him fully, holding nothing back, even your own person, when many women would have surrendered to distaste and repugnance. You have not abandoned him; you have made the only decision possible."

Now, for the first time in years, Helen had time for some concentrated reading and study. At first the total silence of the house beat on her eardrums. Then she decided to take part of her vacation to read *The Desire of Ages* yet again. She would read an hour in the morning, an hour at noon, and an hour at night. The rest of the time she spent painting the rooms, working in the yard, putting on new screens, stripping the old paint off the kitchen and repainting it, sanding windowsills, and the other thousand and one things that a homeowner must do to keep property at top value.

The Desire of Ages became her friend. The characters in the book, especially her Saviour, seemed to be spending the days with her. She would read, then reread and mark. One day she almost spoke aloud as a strong impression came to her mind. "All along, Jesus was trying to prepare His disciples for His death," she realized. "He was always trying to change their ideas of what His coming really was about. And yet they still did not see, did not understand." The parallel became clear to her. "All these decades, He has been trying to get all of us as Adventists to see what He really wants us to become, and we haven't seen it, haven't grasped it."

In some of her other reading, a sentence from *In Heavenly Places* literally leaped from the page into her mind: "The highest honor that can be conferred upon human beings, be they young or old, rich or poor, is to be permitted to lift up the oppressed, to comfort the feeble-minded."—Page 173. For a brief moment, she felt exalted, uplifted, chosen for a special work.

That small period of time would never be anything but one of the most precious of Helen's memories, though nothing external was visible as a reminder.

Throughout her lifetime Helen had been disappointed in herself many times. It seemed to her that she did not stay on an even keel emotionally as much as she would like to have done. Even though the psychiatrist whom she consulted assured her that the trials she was forced to cope with accounted for much of her mood swings, she was not totally satisfied that this was the entire answer.

At about this time, when the medical field began to publicize the work of endocrinologists, Helen decided to make one last attempt to find out more about her physical manifestations. As she gave her history to the endocrinologist's office nurse, Helen exclaimed, almost in desperation,

"Why do I sometimes dissolve into tears under pressure? Why do I feel shaky? Why am I sometimes so depressed? Why is my mouth often like cotton?"

Tests revealed that Helen bordered on diabetes.

"Well, at last I have found that there really is something physically wrong!" she exclaimed to her doctor, who put her on a high-protein, low-carbohydrate, and no-sugar diet, and biweekly shots for several years. As the weeks and months progressed, the symptoms that had been so troublesome to Helen disappeared. Now she could face what must be faced with more courage and stability. (Her friends thought she had *always* shown courage.)

In talking with a friend, Helen remembered the diet of her youth. "During the depression we always ate lots of starches and sweets because they were filling. And when Stan and I were married, we had such a tiny amount of money for food that again I filled us up on that sort of thing."

Her friend chuckled. "And don't forget, Helen, that in those days a woman's homemaking skills were judged on the basis of what kind of cakes and pies she could turn out!"

Helen agreed. "I was determined not to be a failure, and so I really worked on that aspect of cooking. And to think it was literally poison to me—and probably to my family!"

With her simple, nourishing food and more tranquillity in her home, Helen began to feel much better physically. But her newfound peace was hard-won. After Stan had been in Simi Valley for only two weeks, he begged to come home just for the weekend. Helen's tender heart could not say No, though her better judgment issued warning after warning. Sure enough, as soon as he was in his home, he announced that he *would not* return to Simi.

"But you asked to go there, Stan dear," Helen reminded him.

Her words were of no avail. He would not listen. He was in a deep depression, probably as a partial result of drugs given him to lessen the incessant twitching and near-convulsing. One minute he was loud and uncontrollable; five minutes later he would be unreachable, sunk in despair.

Nonetheless, Helen could not take him back in his frame of mind. "You hate me!" he screamed at her. "Nobody loves me! Why can't I die?"

She tried to soothe him. "Let's see how things go if you stay here," she told him. That night her prayer season was long. "Her" text came again to her mind: "Though he slay me, yet will I trust in him."

On Monday morning, as she prepared to go to her office, she became aware that a storm was brewing. Sure enough, Stan went completely out of control, crying uncontrollably. She could not leave him alone. He could never be left alone again.

In panic, she wondered how she would get him into the car for the sad trip—the long trip—back to Simi Valley Hospital up the coast. She must phone her office, must explain, though she shrank from others' knowing the full extent of Stan's illness. It was so humiliating for him, so crushing. Then, after all was done, she sat down with him and talked slowly and calmly. Gradually the tension left his body. Gradually the storm subsided.

"And so, Stan darling, don't you think it's best for me to take you back to Simi?" she finally asked him.

This time he was docile.

This time when she left him the tears could not be held back.

At times some of the old questions that Helen had wrestled with for so long came back to haunt her. Why had her entire life, with the exception of only a few years, been spent in taking care of the sick? Had she failed to listen to the Lord so long ago when she prayed that He would guide in her answer to Stan's marriage proposal? Had she been so starry-eyed and dazzled that she was in no frame of mind to listen to the still, small voice?

Sensibly, now, she was more able to push these

questions aside. From the viewpoint of so many years, she couldn't affort to waste her energy in regrets. One day at her typewriter, when the questioning seemed especially intense, suddenly a tremendous realization hit her. If she hadn't married Stan, there wouldn't have been Jacquee and Margie and the grandchildren! There might have been other children and other grandchildren, but not these, so inexpressibly dear. Give them up? Never. "I guess I thought all this time no matter whom I had married, I'd still have had these human beings for my own." She smiled to herself, the joke too private to share with anyone else.

A trial more difficult to settle "once and for all" was her loneliness and isolation. She was not single. But she was not really married. She couldn't find a place where she really fit in. In spite of the much-vaunted "women's lib," it seemed to Helen that everything in the world moved in pairs, much like the animals who had gone obediently into Noah's ark. She felt at times as though she'd suffered some sort of amputation that made her an object of revulsion. Yet she told herself again and again that it was all her imagination, that if she were more intelligent, more perceptive, she could find a social niche for herself.

Actually, though, it would have been next to impossible. There were the four long workdays, the Friday half-day, and the afternoon with cleaning, cooking, washing, ironing, and household errands to be taken care of. Almost automatically she fell into the routine of preparing food on Friday that could be packed as a good lunch for Sabbath. On Sabbath morning she would get up early and be out on the freeways for the long trip up the coast to Simi Valley Hospital. Surprisingly, Stan, under constant medication that seemed still able to control his behavior, usually was dressed properly and waiting for her to take him to church.

At first the walk into the church and down the aisle was a torment to Helen, for Stan's sake. By now she suffered from a hearing loss severe enough to make it necessary for her to sit right at the front if she was to get anything out of the service. Otherwise she and Stan could have slipped quietly and inconspicuously into one of the rear pews. She had been accustomed to his changed appearance herself, and at times felt she was resigned to the fact that others would stare at him, but from time to time the realization struck her anew. Her once-handsome, eloquent Stan, singer of sweet songs, immaculate, perceptive, refined—who was this stranger at Simi Valley bearing his name? She wanted to shout to church members, "I wish you could have known him before; I wish you could have known him before!"

But of course she did not. She accepted with grief the fact that no one could feel comfortable with the two of them, because of Stan's disability. One thing she could do and did: she dressed him beautifully when he was in public. Never did she stint on his clothes, even if her own were worn a long time and were plain. She derived considerable solace from the pretty shirts and ties she bought him, from the attractive dress suit she always managed to have in good order for him.

After the service the two of them would make their way out of the church, returning the timid greetings of members who made an effort to show at least a modicum of concern. Then into the car and to one of several spots where Stan could enjoy the picnic lunch. The ritual became established. Church, lunch, then a ride. He sat beside her, unresponsive, gazing from the window while she chattered, vainly trying to interest him, trying to penetrate the secrets of his dying mind. She had learned, from long years of practice, to recognize the signs of overfatigue in his mannerisms. She had learned to be alert to danger signals so that she could get him back to the hospital in time.

Though he seemed so unresponsive, the leave-taking bruised her heart each week. He would not let her take him to his room. He would stand in the doorway of the hospital, straining his eyes, gazing at her and the car as long as they were in sight. She would look back over her shoulder and he would still be standing there, alone, shaking convulsively, leaning against the wall. The hot tears would roll down her cheeks. Sometimes she wondered why, after a while, tears do not disappear—just dry up, like the desert. But they did not.

Always alert to hobbies that would provide her with something to think about, Helen enrolled in a class in pottery-making and produced a few beautiful things. The whole process of working with clay on a potter's wheel so intrigued her that she resolved to have her own wheel one day and see whether she could come up with some kind of original pottery. For the moment, though, extra money (if any) had to be applied to Stan's bills. And there was never enough time to keep up with creative clamorings.

As soon as Stan had returned from Chicago, Helen had set about taking out whatever health insurance she could get for him. After he had been diagnosed as so seriously ill, no company would then take him. However, when the facts of his case were finally established, she began to receive some medical aid from the General Conference. Unfortunately, nothing in this line could ever be enough as his expenses mounted.

Medicare and other small insurance paid only a few weeks at Simi. Helen herself managed the rest, how she would never know, as the weeks and months rolled by. When she would come to the point of desperation, somehow a bit of extra money presented itself.

Then she was called by the hospital administrator. "Mrs. Jefferson," he said, "we have decided that we really can't keep your husband here any longer. He doesn't need the total care that we are giving—in time he will, but for now we need the bed."

Helen felt the familiar panic start in the pit of her stomach. She had thought that finally her problem was solved. "What shall I do—where can I take him?" she begged.

He thought for a moment. "You know," he told her

slowly, "I think he could still manage for a while in an intermediate facility. He needs to be in a 'Board and Care' facility."

"That is the first time I've ever heard of that kind of place," Helen told him. "Can you explain it to me?"

The administrator told her that these facilities, few though they were, took patients who could not be left alone but who did not need total nursing care. But he did not know of any place to suggest in southern California. Helen was again up against a brick wall, but now she had learned to turn to her one unfailing Friend and Counselor.

"Lord, where shall I put Stan now?" she begged that night on her knees by her bed.

The answer came. Her dear friend Etta Blacker, upon hearing of the new problem, said, "Helen, I heard that there's a new place opened about half a mile from Glendale Adventist Hospital. It's called Casa Bonita. Why don't you go to see it?"

Hardly daring to hope, Helen phoned for an appointment. Her heart in her mouth, she drove up to the beautiful new building, was shown through the nice new rooms, and, holding her breath, asked the price. She was almost giddy with relief when she found it was much lower than hospital care—and her cup was full of joy when the administrator told her they had a vacancy. They would take Stan.

When she drove the long freeways to Simi, packed Stan's clothes, and made arrangements for his transfer, he was like a child. "Will I like it there, Mommy?" he asked her trustingly. She turned her face away to hide the sudden tears.

Later, after Stan's death, Helen would learn that Stan had still possessed enough of his old sweet and loving nature to endear himself to many of the patients at Simi Valley. When he was not suffering the extreme manifestations of his disease, he tried to encourage others and lift their spirits. Thinking of the pathos of his attempts to continue—even in his extremity—vestiges of his ministry, Helen again felt the old familiar lump in her throat.

Later, at Fillmore, it would be the same. When he was able he was, they told her, an "inspiration."

Helen would wonder whether his embarrassment when he was with her, his reluctance to let her know all his degradations, caused him to be less a man with her than he was with his peer group of sufferers who probably accepted one another with compassion.

Had she failed him? Had she appeared judgmental? She hadn't felt that way. She still loved him, loved just to touch him, caress his forehead, trying to let him know she cared and suffered with him.

Now he was closer to home; she could drop in and see him evenings if he was in a mood to be with her. This varied from day to day. If his mood was one of deep depression, it was hopeless to try to talk with him. If he were highly excitable, her presence might push him over the brink into lack of control. But he seemed more contented during these months. Sometimes he would ask her to take his soiled clothes home. "I want you to wash my clothes for me, Mommy," he would beg, and she would take them, knowing that the laundry at Casa Bonita was completely adequate but glad to give him this small evidence of her love.

As Helen's birthday approached, Stan walked to the nearest Robinson's Department Store, which carried beautiful merchandise. He bought her—very proudly, with money she gave him—a quart of Jean Naté bath lotion. Helen always kept money in his wallet, even knowing that it might be stolen from him by other patients. She felt he was entitled to this evidence of personhood and self-respect. She was afraid for him ever to be alone in a crowd, but his purchases were intensely important to him.

At Christmas Stan solemnly repeated the buying trip. "Well, I'll never lack for bath lotion," Helen chuckled to herself, her natural sense of humor asserting itself.

The year 1974 was one ringed in black on Helen's mental

calendar. Somehow she had fallen into a depression that, try though she might to escape, kept her imprisoned. The devil never let her rest from trials of one sort or another, particularly in the realm of human relations. On one Sabbath she would never forget, she took Stan to a church they hadn't attended during the year he was a patient at Simi Valley. The wife of one of the deacons approached her when she was at some distance from Stan.

"Well," the woman said airily, looking at Stan, "it occurs to me that maybe he really was sick, the way you claimed!"

Helen could not believe her ears. She stood frozen. Could any professed Christian be so cold, so rude, so calloused? Could the woman not see the tragedy of her and Stan's lives? Did she have no heart at all?

Muttering something, Helen turned away, took Stan's arm, escorted him into the sanctuary, and sat down with him, fighting back the tears. The encounter had brought back all the old sick feelings of shame and disgrace that she had battled during the years when Stan had left home and his illness had not been diagnosed. She realized now that some people would never believe he was ill when he left; they would prefer to believe that he had "disgraced" himself and his family.

She had been sure Stan was still capable enough mentally, especially in the early years, to know that church members looked down on him. She had feared that unchristian cruelty might keep him from ever finding his way back to God. Yet God had overruled, and Stan had been rebaptized.

Sometimes it had been difficult for her to attend Adventist services. She had concluded that one of the great benefits from her classwork was that the class members in her painting, china painting, and pottery classes were non-Adventist. She did not feel self-conscious or strange or singled out. But she wondered whether she would ever again have the marvelous feeling of "belonging" that had been so much a part of her life when Stan was a successful young minister. Perhaps she never would.

The weeks dragged as Helen wrestled with her natural resentments. She spent more time in prayer, more time in Bible study, often waking at four in the morning. Sometimes it was hard to accept "Though he slay me . . ."

Now Stan entered a period of relative tranquillity, and Helen was able to establish a new routine with him. On summer Fridays, when sunset was late, she would pick him up at Casa Bonita and take him to a restaurant for a simple, inexpensive meal. He had begged and begged to do this—somehow it represented to him the last link with "the good life." When Margie heard of the plan, she remonstrated on the phone, "But Mother, what if he should become uncontrollable? What if——"

Helen interrupted her. "I've thought of all those possibilities, Margie dear," she said, "but I refuse to surrender your father to the pit of his disease until I absolutely have to."

Margie was still apprehensive. "Won't people notice his problems and stare?" she asked fearfully.

"They may, but I'm used to that. And I'll take him to little restaurants where people aren't expected to be perfect," Helen assured her. Often she saw other handicapped people being taken for a brief period of pleasure. What a suffering world it was!

And so Stan looked forward to his summer Friday nights or his winter Saturday nights with the longing of a child. The "Casa Bonita Years," as Helen would later think of them, were sadly happy, if that word could ever be used for his situation. He had a room with a beautiful view of Glendale Adventist Hospital and the majestic hills rimming the valley. He began listening for Helen's "toot" as she circled the hospital; he would be waiting at the front door.

Sometimes Helen would fantasize that Stan was convalescing from a long illness and that in due time he would return to her whole and sane again. But she could not hold the fantasy long, for he would begin to twitch more violently, would lose the thread of the conversation, would talk wildly—and then the sickening realization would be borne in again on her that it was a sorrow with only one possible ending.

If only they had had another couple willing to give their time to spend an occasional Friday night or Sabbath afternoon! If only they were not always so alone, so alone!

One difference that became obvious was Stan's dissolution of his ties with home. He no longer asked to be brought home. He did not refer to their house, though Helen chattered brightly, telling him everything she had done. When she would ask him whether he wanted to be taken home for a visit, he mumbled incoherently. Tired and strained as she was, she accepted what she could not change. In the peace and privacy of her home, her nerves could regenerate for whatever the future held.

One day when her mind seemed to ache and her heart was so heavy that she could not find any rays of light, Helen suddenly decided to sit down and list her hobbies—both the ones she now pursued and those she might like in the future, if ever time presented itself. Just the listing was fun.

Gardening outdoors and houseplants indoors. (Some of her houseplants were a couple of years old; they were like friends.) Knitting and crocheting, especially afghans. (The colors were so satisfying.) Piano. Organ. (Someday she planned to be a better organist.) Reading. Letter writing. Art—watercolors, acrylic, oil, charcoal, pastels, pencil drawings, pen-and-ink drawings. Making scrapbooks, using cloth, lace, ribbon, and wallpaper. Walking. Filing quotations on hand-decorated 4″ x 6″ cards. Flower arranging. Sewing for the grandchildren. (That had been such a joy; it still was.)

The list of happy things broke through the darkness. It became something she did, now and then, mentally. She cataloged a list of her "favorite things."

At the back of her mind was a thought, a tiny thought, that she almost never voiced. It was this: God is the Creator. He is the Healer. He can work any miracle He chooses. If He chose, He could heal Stan. Once in a while she would dream, briefly, that it might happen.

And so life had fallen into a kind of routine—when a new cataclysm hit Helen's life. After much study, discussion, and investigation, the Pacific Union Conference voted to move its headquarters from Glendale to Thousand Oaks, about fifty miles north of Glendale—a very hard fifty miles of driving on crowded, high-speed freeways.

Helen was secretary to the president of the Pacific Union.

"What will I do?" she asked him.

"Don't worry. With your skills, you can easily get a job in one of the other institutions here in Glendale, such as the Southern California Conference office or the Adventist Health Services or the Voice of Prophecy. But wouldn't you like to move to Thousand Oaks and continue as my secretary?" he asked.

Helen had had to make so many decisions during the past years that for a moment she seemed frozen, immobile.

"I must think and pray," she told him.

Each time she prayed, it seemed to her that there was a wall between Glendale and Thousand Oaks and that it was black on the Glendale side and sunny and bright on the Thousand Oaks side. Was the Lord trying to tell her something? But what would she do with Stan if she moved there? She felt that she should apply at one or two of the Glendale offices, which she did, but nothing was available that fitted her skills. She began driving to Thousand Oaks on the busy freeway every Sunday, looking for a house. Each week, it seemed to her, prices were higher.

Helen sat down and figured. "With spiraling inflation, I think I can get at least $35,000 out of the little house I bought for $19,500. Of course, I've put some money and a lot of work into it!" Then her heart would fail her. She loved that little house, every square inch of it. What a haven it had been, after the dark, ugly apartment! It was like a shell, holding her safe and secure.

Finally, in November, she reluctantly made a $200 down payment on a house soon to be built on a road that had not even been cut yet, in Newbury Park, a few minutes' drive from Thousand Oaks. The lots were not even staked off, so she couldn't get a clear picture of how large they would be. But the house, with carpet and appliances, would sell for $41,500. She could not hope to get anything for a lower figure. With her heart in her mouth, she wondered whether she really could get what she needed from the La Crescenta house and whether, at her age, she would be successful in applying for a mortgage. But she had never lacked courage where financial decisions were concerned. She had even managed again to save a few hundred dollars, in spite of Stan's bills.

CHAPTER 16

The Story Ends

IN THE spring of 1976 the office staff at the Pacific Union Conference were told that the building in Thousand Oaks would be completed in June and the move would be made. Now Helen had to burn her bridges. She contacted a real-estate agent and confided her needs.

"I'm having to pay $41,250 for the new house, but I don't suppose I could get that for this house," she sighed.

On a Friday afternoon in April she and the agent sat down to talk. After touring the house, the agent exclaimed, "Why, Mrs. Jefferson, this is a marvelous house! I know it will sell! When can I bring people to see it?"

Helen tried to explain about the Sabbath. "From sundown Friday until sundown Saturday it can't be shown," she concluded.

"Well, a week from Sunday I'd like to keep the house open all day," she told Helen, who agreed with alacrity. Already John had come from the Midwest, had helped her paper the bathroom and put new Solarian linoleum in both the bath and the kitchen. She had labored over the yard. It was beautiful with the springtime flowers. The house was as ready as it would ever be for prospective buyers.

When the phone rang at six o'clock on Saturday night, Helen couldn't believe her ears. "Can I bring some clients by? We have five offers on your house!"

Helen was speechless. "But people haven't even seen it!"

The agent chuckled. "Well, they've seen the outside of it. Haven't you noticed the cars driving up and down your street today and slowing down in front of your house?"

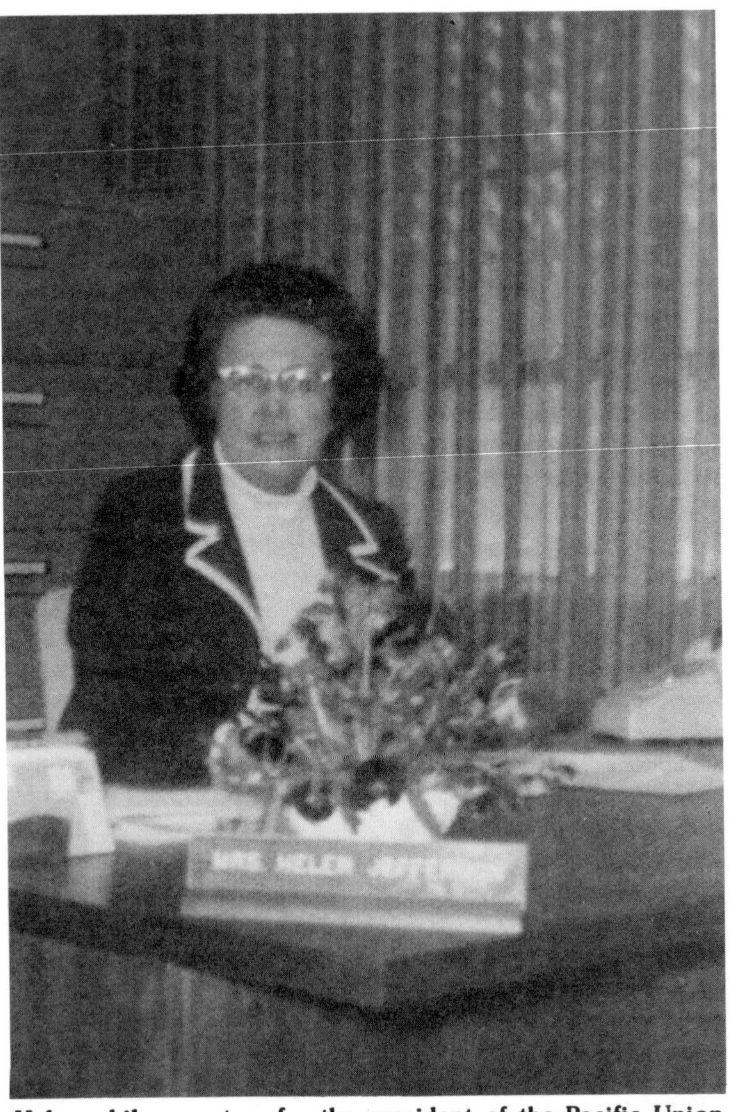

Helen while secretary for the president of the Pacific Union Conference.

Helen threw the door open when the prospective buyers started arriving. She was sure that one set after another would find that the house wasn't what they had visualized—that it didn't, after all, meet their needs.

She was wrong. Five checks were offered. All five couples begged for the house.

"What can I do?" she implored the agent. "I want to be fair."

After thinking for a moment, the broker said, "Why don't you suggest that whoever will meet the price of your new place gets this house, and then see what happens?"

Helen breathed a silent prayer. "Lord, please guide me and help me to be fair and not to make any mistakes," she pleaded. Her prayer was answered. One couple was willing to match the amount of the new house. The broker assured Helen that her La Crescenta house was an enormous bargain at that price, that she need have no fears that she had "gouged" someone. And so the papers were signed.

Helen moved into her new house in Newbury Park at the end of May, expecting that the office would be ready in June. Now she had a "reverse commuting" to do, leaving the house between six and six-thirty each morning to get to the Glendale office, and not arriving home until after seven at night. Each drive had to be done at the heaviest time of traffic and against the rising or setting sun, always blinding.

She realized immediately that she could not take the drive back on Sabbath to be with Stan. Her nerves were frayed and torn from all the work she had done in the moving process. Before she had moved she had taken Stan to see the new house. She had tried to explain all the business dealings and the enormous blessing that the Lord had wrought.

"Why, honey, I didn't have to worry even one day about whether or not the house would sell," she told him. "Isn't God good to us? Don't we have a lot to be thankful for?"

He mumbled his assent. When it was time to sign the papers for the new house, she took him with her and insisted that both signatures appear. "I want you to know that this is your home just as much as the other one was," she told him. To herself she thought, If, by the greatest miracle, he should ever be himself again, I would want him to know that he had been treated with dignity and respect.

Not only did Helen feel that God had provided a buyer for her house but when the daily commuting was too much for her to continue on Sabbath, God seemed to stabilize Stan to the point where she stopped at Casa Bonita on her way home from the office on Friday, packed his suitcase, drove him to the new house in Thousand Oaks, and kept him for the weekend. She had not done this for some time. The first time she attempted it, her heart was in her mouth.

June. July. August. September. The daily commuting was taking its toll. Weekends were strenuous; she could not leave Stan alone for any length of time. Then, in October, the union office was finally ready; the move was made. Helen had only a short drive each day from her home to the office, along a back road with a lovely rural setting.

By this time her new house had been the object of a great deal of mirth, Helen laughing loudest and longest of all. When she discovered that the clay soil was absolutely hopeless, she ran across some advertising that praised the idea of using sludge for fertilizer. The advertisement went on at great length to describe how miraculous the sludge was—you would have to force grass *not* to grow in it! Helen lay awake thinking of the joys of a lawn, finally. No more struggles with the hard clay. "Maybe I ought to get sixteen cubic yards of sludge" was her last drowsy thought, but on awaking, a voice seemed to say, "Helen, eight yards would be enough." Later on, she would be sure an angel had spoken to her, for when the eight yards were delivered, it almost swamped both yard and house.

Learnedly Helen explained about the sludge to her office friends. "Actually, it's nitrohumous. It's what the sewage-disposal plants have—they run it through and pulverize it."

Helen didn't mention the "perfume" of the huge pile of sludge.

When finally she had hauled load after load around the yard and planted her seeds, it was as though the plants sprang up overnight. There was, however, one problem. To her horror, Helen saw tomato plants springing up all over her yard, front and back. Neighbors and friends began coming by to see the latest in the saga of "Helen's Tomato Patch."

"What in the world has happened? What will I do?" she cried to a friendly neighbor.

"Well," he chuckled, "I don't think anyone told you that a sewage-disposal plant doesn't kill tomato seeds. And what you can do is pluck up every tomato plant *by hand!*"

Between the hours of backbreaking labor with the tomato plants and enduring the smell of the sludge and its dreadful black color, which persisted for months, Helen wished heartily that she had never seen the advertisement.

"Don't anyone ever say 'sludge' to me again!" she laughed at the office.

Now that the house was somewhat settled and the yard was taking shape (albeit slowly), she had to restudy Stan's situation. She did not want him so far from her. She felt he needed the reassurance of being near her; she dreaded the long drive each Sabbath on the freeway.

But nothing seemed to open up. This section of the coast was not as thickly settled at that time as other sections. She ran down every lead, phoned every convalescent home. No vacancies. She began praying fervently again. Had she made a mistake in moving to the Thousand Oaks vicinity? Had she mistaken the Lord's leading? Should she have made a greater effort to get a job in Glendale?

When all seemed insoluble, she heard of a little Spanish lady only two miles away who had five patients in her home. Helen raced to see her. After she explained Stan's condition, "Sally," as she would come to know her, thought for a few moments.

"Yes, Mrs. Jefferson, I will take him if he will be cooperative," she announced.

Helen felt a small stirring of uneasiness. One could not predict Stan's mood and attitude at any given time. "He has been cooperative for the past year and perhaps he will continue" was her honest answer. "But he will continue to fail."

Suddenly Stan seemed to be drifting downward rapidly. When she told him of the new plans, he seemed listless, disoriented, as though it did not concern him.

"Stan darling," she urged, "I think you will like this place. Sally is such a lovely person. There are only five other patients, so it will be like being in a home again. And I will be able to see you every weekend and some evenings and—well, it will just be nice all the way around!"

And so in January he was ensconced in Sally's little "halfway house."

At first he was cooperative. He ate what Sally prepared for him; she always tried to give him the things he liked. He kept himself clean. But as the months went by, Sally began phoning Helen at work.

"I can't do anything with him today," she would complain. "He has wet himself and won't let me change his clothes."

Helen would have to leave her office, drive to the home, reason with Stan, and try to effect a reconciliation between him and Sally. Sometimes she would succeed. Sometimes she would not. Sometimes he would be almost violent, his whole body racked and shaking.

A few more months passed. The calls from Sally continued. "He throws his food on the floor. He has lost control of his bodily functions. I am not equipped to handle this kind of thing. I did not realize from your description of his condition that this was how it would be," Sally stated, her voice becoming more and more accusatory.

Helen tried to explain that she had not deliberately

deceived Sally, that Stan had not been like this at Casa Bonita. "His disease has taken a decided downward turn," she declared.

Sally was unmoved. "I don't think I can handle him much longer," she insisted.

During this period Jacquee was forced to undergo very serious spinal-disk surgery. In August, after years of intense suffering, she finally made the decision to have the surgery. But she was terrified. By now she had had so many surgeries, had suffered so much.

"When you get home from the hospital I'm coming to Sacramento to take care of you," Helen told her on the phone. "Be brave; I know the Lord will bless the surgeon."

Helen took her vacation as Jacquee's nurse. But when, after weeks of intense suffering, Jacquee suddenly improved dramatically, it was all worthwhile. Helen had grieved over the long, long incision down her daughter's slender back. As she thought of the scalpels cutting into the flesh, her heart quailed.

Now she must—as soon as she returned home—again face the question: What to do with Stan?

Her heart ached when she saw him on her visit to Sally's after the weeks in Sacramento. When he stood, his toes turned blue. Coronary insufficiency. His humanity was now becoming almost totally obscured. The cruel, cruel disease was robbing him of all that he had been, all that he could have been. Silently she wondered, Why can't he die peacefully and be through with his sufferings? Why must he go on and on and on like this?

In an effort to break through his clouded mind, she went shopping for him and bought a beautiful beige suit, a new pair of shoes, a beautiful dark-brown shirt with a matching orange-and-brown tie, and a blue shirt with a blue-and-maroon tie.

She could not know that she would one day bury him in the beautiful beige suit.

In January, 1978, Sally told Helen that Stan would have to be moved. "I feel terribly sorry, but he can hardly be gotten out of his bed. He will eat almost nothing." And then Sally went on to describe other manifestations of the bitter disease that Helen could hardly bear to hear.

As she prayed that night Helen remembered that earlier in Stan's long illness, the administrator of Ventura Estates (not far from her present home) had said to her, "Helen, if ever you want to put Stan here, you had better fill out an application blank and have us keep it on file, because our waiting list is so long." Helen had thought this to be very good counsel and had done so. Now she felt that perhaps this would be an answer. When she drove to Ventura Estates and showed them her copy of the application, turned in years before, they had the matching copy.

"But we don't have a men's ward at the moment—and there is simply no opening for a man," she was told.

Helen felt the old familiar panic return.

"What shall I do?" she cried.

"There's a facility in Fillmore that I think might fit your needs," the administrator told her. "That's about an hour's drive from here."

Immediately Helen had a mental picture of the long trips on the freeways, the calls from the nurses when Stan was uncontrollable and she so far away. But as she studied and investigated, she found that Fillmore had to be the choice.

"How can I face all that paper work again?" she groaned inwardly. "To say nothing of phone calls and letters to the doctors in the new place and the dragging of all Stan's medical records and the notifying of the insurance company and Medicare and all the rest!" Helen never seemed able to see the doctors in person. They were remote, inaccessible.

Quickly she mentally took herself by the scruff of the neck and gave herself a shaking. "Stop that!" she urged herself. "That's about enough of that kind of whining. Of course you can get it all done. You've certainly had enough experience!"

But the paper work wasn't the worst. Stan did not want to stay at Sally's, but he was violently antagonistic toward being taken to Fillmore.

"You can take me there, but I will never walk!" he threatened, and that was exactly what he did. From the day he entered Fillmore, he refused to walk.

Even this was not the worst. He began holding his breath as long as he possibly could, hoping that he would die. Helen tried to reason with him.

"Stan dear, a person can't hold his breath long enough to commit suicide," she told him. "If you become unconscious, you will start breathing again."

When he found she was right, he went into periods of screaming, hour after hour, until he was exhausted, as were the hospital personnel who tried to soothe him.

Then he refused all food. He wasted away to a shriveled form curled in solitary anguish in his bed. Finally Helen persuaded him to eat a few mouthfuls, but from then on his consumption of food was below the starvation level. Early in his diagnosis she had been told that eventually he would have to be fed with tubes—he would not be able to swallow.

Now Sabbaths were a horror, for Helen would get up early, have her devotions and her breakfast, go to church, and then be on the freeways to Fillmore. All afternoon she sat by Stan's bed, feeding him, trying to talk with him, trying to make him feel her love and concern. But he was very, very far gone.

"Girls, I can't endure seeing Daddy suffer like this," she told her daughters on a long-distance phone call. "Oh, if God would just let him go to his rest peacefully! The Lord knows that he is not responsible for the way he is. How horrible that he continues to live and suffer, suffer, suffer."

"That's the terrible thing about Huntington's disease," Margie replied sadly. "The victim just seems to go on and on in the most awful torment. Maybe it won't be much longer, though."

An added trial came in the form of a severe rainstorm that washed out roads and bridges. For two or three weeks the roads to the Fillmore Hospital were closed. Helen felt panicked again. What if Stan should die? What if the hospital needed her?

Moreover, in June both Margie and Jacquee made trips to see him. Horrified, they gazed at the bedsores on his ears, his head, his shoulders, his elbows, and his hips. There seemed not to be one part of his body that was not an open sore, not one part that was not constantly moving and jerking. All the hair was worn from his head.

"Why isn't his medication calming him?" Margie demanded, her medical background asserting itself.

Helen phoned the doctor.

"Oh, we've taken him off his medications" was the reply.

Helen was angry. "Why?" she demanded.

"I don't remember why," he said offhandedly.

Helen replied, "You did not get permission from me. I insist that you give him his medication again immediately. He cannot live like this. I will not have it."

After the resumption of calming medications, the sores healed and his hair grew back. But Jacquee and Margie's last visit with him was forever clouded by that agonizing situation in June of 1978.

Just when Helen felt that she could not cope with anything more, a small light broke through. She received a call from the administrator of Ventura Estates.

"We're opening up another men's ward—we'll have a bed for your husband if you want it," he told her.

Helen could hardly believe that God had worked for her so lovingly once again. The care at Ventura Estates was well known to be superlative. The hospital was just a few miles from her house.

"Oh, thank you, thank you; you will never know what this means. But how will we move him? He isn't walking, you know."

The administrator thought for a moment. "We'll send our station wagon" was his suggestion, so Stan was moved in early September.

"Mrs. Jefferson," the head nurse said gently, when Helen was through with all the paper work again, "we have just weighed your husband. He weighs only sixty-four pounds."

Helen felt the lump in her throat. She had known that he had wasted away almost to a skeleton, but she had not realized that his weight was that of a small child.

Seeing her distress, the nurse said, "We'll see whether we can't get him to eat more. Don't think about it too much; we'll take over from here."

What blessed words! What comfort! They were true to their word. When Stan died, he weighed about 120 pounds.

Things did seem a great deal better at Ventura Estates. Realizing this, Helen's mind was calm, her nerves less taut. The attendants really cared about the patients. It was obvious in their manner, their method of addressing the poor souls in their care, the sparkling cleanliness of the institution, the good food. Far gone as he was, Stan responded. His outbursts were less frequent. But now he did not always know her when she came to see him. She would find him lying in his bed, staring emptily into space. Sometimes he would converse with her; sometimes he would not.

"He used to like television," she said to herself. "Maybe that could arouse him just a little." And so she brought his TV set from home, and the handyman hung it on the wall where he could see it. She wondered whether or not he ever watched it. She could not get a response from him when she asked. One day, however, the wife of another patient in the ward said to her, "He watches the television set a lot; the nurses turn it on for him and he seems to enjoy it."

During that last year, though, he became totally helpless. He could not even give himself a drink of water. He was a lump, a stone, pitiful, tragic, unmoving.

Sometimes, alone in her house, thinking of Stan, now a

stranger, alone and afraid, a captive of the vicious invading force in his body, Helen thought that her own heart would break with grief. When these times came, God seemed always to provide a comfort, a surcease. On one occasion, she bought a Marilyn Cotton record and as she listened she was convinced that one song was meant for her and her alone. How could it be any other way, with such a title? She played it over and over, memorizing the words, humming it to herself as the days passed.

Is your life full of heartache and sadness?
Are your dreams all shattered and torn?
There is One who through mercy and suffering
For you every sorrow has borne.

He's the healer of broken hearts.
He'll mend your shattered dreams.
He'll pick up the threads of your broken life
And weave them together again.
To your soul He'll bring peace and joy;
A friend in need He'll be.
The healer of broken hearts
Is Jesus of Galilee.

Do the threads of your life seems so tangled
That you wish you had never been born?
There is One who is willing to help you;
He knows every sorrow you've borne.

He's the healer of broken hearts.
He'll mend your shattered dreams.
He'll pick up the threads of your broken life
And weave them together again.
To your soul He'll bring peace and joy;
A friend in need He'll be
The healer of broken hearts
Is Jesus of Galilee.

Marilyn's incomparable, silvery soprano became a lifeline.

The days no longer had meaning for Stan. He did not know one day from another. Each Sabbath when Helen came and spent the long afternoon, weeping bitterly as she returned home, she began to feel that a Sunday visit would be just as good. She was starved for more church relationships, so long denied her. And so she began attending more church activities, mingling, making more friends—and spending every Sunday afternoon with Stan.

But it was a comfort to her to realize that lovely Sabbath music was brought into all the wards of the Ventura Estates Hospital. Perhaps Stan would recognize it—somehow, someway.

On the last Sabbath of Stan's life, Helen had been invited out to a friend's home for lunch—a rare and prized occasion for her. Then one of the group suggested that they drive the hour and a half to La Crescenta to hear the speaker in an effort being held.

"Well—that's kind of a long drive," Helen commented, doubtfully.

"To us Californians it's nothing," they all laughed.

Secure in the knowledge that she would spend the next day at Stan's bedside, Helen went along, reveling in the fellowship of others, in the beauty of the day, in the surcease from care and anxiety.

When she returned to her house at about eleven o'clock that night, her phone was ringing.

"Mrs. Jefferson, I'm afraid it's bad news," a voice said. "Your husband is having trouble breathing. You'd better come at once. We've been trying to contact you all afternoon and evening."

Her heart in her mouth, Helen drove the short distance, walked through the darkness into the building, and into Stan's ward.

The figure on the bed, emaciated and pitiful, obviously was choking with fluid and phlegm in the lungs. From her extensive reading about Huntington's disease, Helen assumed that he had contracted pneumonia. She knew that his muscles would not be sufficiently strong for him to clear his lungs. All afternoon they had been suctioning him out, the nurse told her, to keep him alive until Helen could be contacted.

Helen started talking to him. "Stan dearest, I'm here. Do you know that?" she asked tenderly.

There was no response from the suffering form. But Helen knew that somewhere in the darkness enclosing him, Stan might still hear her voice. He might still receive comfort from her presence.

"Daddy, I will never leave you," she told him, pressing his limp hand.

At one point he tried to make a little sound in response to her voice. Her heart almost broke as the poor, suffering creature tried to communicate with her.

"I love you, sweetheart," she told him, tears raining down her cheeks. "I always have."

She slipped away briefly to phone Jacquee and Margie. "We're coming on the first plane," they told her through their tears.

Then she noticed a change in his body. Always his muscles had been so tight, so contracted, that she could barely move his arms. He was always locked in a vise of torment. Now when she picked up his arm, it was soft, flexible. As death approached, at last the terrible invader of his body was himself forced to relinquish his suffering victim.

Midnight came. Stan's breathing became lighter, more shallow. Helen continued to hold his hand, to talk to him, to bathe his face with a cold cloth, to kiss his high, beautiful forehead, still unchanged.

One o'clock came. Now he breathed so lightly that she had to bend down to be sure that it was not her imagination.

Two o'clock. She prayed over and over, "Lord, Stan is Your child. When he had his mind, he loved You with all his heart. You know what he has suffered. Please, please make his dying easy. Please forgive him for the things he could not help. Please forgive him for all his sins and let him go to sleep in Your love, like a trusting child, and when You come, bring him forth in radiant health!"

Then the faint, tentative breaths ceased. Stan's face seemed to smooth out into peaceful, tranquil lines.

It was over. The long, cruel, tragic story had ended. It was February 25, 1979.

As Helen sat beside his bed, holding his hand for the last time, just the two of them together, alone, suddenly she was back in memory in the little church in Reno, forty years before—so long ago. It was their wedding day. Her tall, dark-eyed, handsome groom was beside her. Ahead were the years of early-married struggles, the lack of money, the hard work. Ahead were Jacquee and Margie and the grandchildren. Ahead were all of the rich experiences of her life. Ahead also were all the broken dreams, the heartaches, which she could not foresee. Most of all, ahead was Stan's tragedy. And her tragedy.

But with a feeling of glorious faith, she realized that God had never forsaken her. He had carried her through every step of the way. He loved her. He loved Stan. He was a God of love. Now the words that she had repeated so often rang with a certainty that almost made her tremble: "Though he slay me, yet will I trust in him."

Smiling softly, she remembered the sweet words of the song her young groom had sung at their wedding reception, words that she had repeated to herself sometimes at night in her loneliness. She closed her eyes, surrendering herself to the memory:

There's a little brown road windin' over the hill
    To a little white cot by the sea.
There's a little green gate, by whose trellis I wait
    While two eyes of blue come smilin' through—at me.

There's a gray lock or two in the brown of your hair;
There's some silver in mine, too, I see;
But in all the long years when the clouds brought their tears,
Those two eyes of blue kept smilin' through—at me.

On some glorious morning, Stan would awake to the sound of God's voice. Her young groom would stand before her in all his handsome strength and consecration. He would smile at her with his brown eyes—and her blue eyes, the eyes he had loved so well, would smile back.

APPENDIX A

Daddy, Whom I Loved *by Jacquee*

DADDY was one of those "one in a million" men. He was always perfectly groomed and totally refined in his appearance. He presented a figure of which I was extremely proud. I remember, as a small child, going places with him and wanting everyone to know *he* was my *father!*

He had many fine qualities. Womanhood, in his opinion, was to be placed on a high pedestal. Mother was treated like a queen, while Margie and I were treated like princesses. We were all spoiled—not so much in monetary things (he would have spoiled us in that area, too, could we have afforded it), but with love, security, and respect.

He loved life, loved young people, and outdoor activities. Some of the happiest memories of my childhood were those "family days" when we would pack a lunch and the four of us would head for the beach, desert, or mountains. It was on these trips that I learned to observe and appreciate the wonders of nature. For instance, the excitement of exploring tide pools for the sea creatures that lived in them, or looking at a small flower blooming in the barren sand, or sitting very quietly with a pair of binoculars waiting for the sight of a rare feathered friend to fly by. Half the fun then was trying to identify each "find" in the guidebooks we would bring with us.

I always felt there was a special closeness between Daddy and me. We seemed to communicate—sometimes without words. We enjoyed many of the same types of things. When I was as young as 7 or 8, I loved orchestra and band concerts. The two of us would go together to hear these concerts on many occasions. A few times he and I went canoeing in the park. We loved boating. Mother and Margie did not share our enthusiasm for this type of sport.

As I grew older and learned to play the piano I would accompany him on his singing engagements. This was a mutually enjoyable time for both of us. Many times at home I would sit at the piano and play while he sang for hours. There are still times when I sit down at the piano and play some of the songs he loved; I can almost hear his clear baritone voice coming over my shoulder.

He was a firm disciplinarian and demanded that we respect both our parents. One night my natural tendency toward stubborn independence came to the fore and I snapped a sassy remark to Mother. Of course Daddy had to administer the necessary punishment. I will never forget that sometime in the middle of the night I roused and felt someone kneeling beside my bed. Dear Daddy was sobbing his heart out. This was the first time in my 14 years I had ever known him to cry. He put his arms around me and gave me a hug—then, through his sobs, he said, "Jacquee, I'm sorry I had to punish you, but you *must* learn to control your temper." I have never forgotten that.

Even through his long illness we seemed to maintain the communication and the "vibes" between us. Even after the insidious disease had just about taken its toll—when he could no longer talk—when he saw me walk up to his bedside, there was that same gleam and twinkle in his eyes that had always been there.

This is the father I will always remember.

APPENDIX B

Remembering Daddy by Margie

WHEN my sister and I were young, we felt a lot of love and security in our home. We felt that we were an important part of our family. Both our parents were warm and kind to us. With Daddy being a minister, his busiest day was the

Sabbath, so he always tried to schedule Sunday as a "family day," if possible, through picnics, trips, and gardening. He baptized both Jacquee and me, and he felt that the church schools were an important part of our upbringing.

When we lived in Glendale and he was in the religious liberty department of the Pacific Union Conference, he was away on trips a great deal, which left Mother with lots of the family decisions to make. It was during this time that Daddy began to make judgments that we questioned. When my sister graduated from Glendale Academy and married so soon afterward, I now feel that if Daddy had been his old self he would have been able to counsel her differently.

With the move to Oakland came a change in schools for me. After a lot of prayer, we chose for me to go to Monterey Bay Academy for my junior and senior years, and I do have many fond memories of my time there and the friends I made. I think it helped me start making decisions on my own while my parents were still close enough to help if I needed them.

Then we moved to Manteca, where my father became the pastor. I remember one day we went out to a lake looking for rocks. We had to select just the right ones—smooth and round and red—for a very attractive walkway that Daddy and I were making in the back yard. Daddy always had Jacquee and me helping him with any project he was working on. He was so patient with us.

Another day I came home and there were three bicycles in the garage, one for each of us (since my sister was married by then and did not live at home). Manteca being a small, flat country town, we got to ride our bikes a lot. How Daddy enjoyed that!

With all the moves my parents made, I still felt that I had security in their love and in my school friends. After Monterey Bay Academy, I attended Pacific Union College for two years, taking pre-nursing. Then I went to Loma Linda School of Nursing. Just about the time I entered nursing, Daddy and

Mother moved to Barstow. It was after my first year of nursing that Mother and I knew something was dreadfully wrong with Daddy; we took him to a doctor at Loma Linda for extensive tests, but nothing specific was found. It was at this point that he decided he wanted to drive a truck.

Before he left home, he had had several large speeding tickets, and finally a doctor from Barstow talked to the judge and explained that Daddy had not been acting rationally, so he was not required to pay the full amounts. But it was so hard to realize he was not thinking clearly and was not himself and that his judgment was no longer reliable.

During the time he was in Chicago we kept writing to him and telling him how much we loved him and how much we missed him. That kept us going. After he left home, Mother went into Glendale Adventist Hospital in a state of shock for several days. I remember seeing her in the hospital crying, but I don't remember how we got the moving van to take our things from Barstow to Glendale. I remember Mother and I looking at apartments in Glendale, but the ones we could afford were so small and so old—it was very depressing to us.

I was very conscious that Daddy had lost most of our money with the frequent moves and his running away. I didn't know how Mother and I could start all over again, but I knew that we had to do it.

It was providential that the junior year of nursing at that time was held at the White Memorial Hospital in Los Angeles, for this meant that I could live in Glendale with Mother and ride with two other nursing students who lived close to the little house we had found. That year Mother and I tried to do everything we could to cheer ourselves up. We took some swimming classes at the YWCA. We went shopping a lot—not "buying" shopping, because we didn't have any money, but "window" shopping, when we looked at all the pretty things.

Daddy came back home to us by the time I graduated from nursing, and we were so happy to have him. We were very thankful that he had not been killed in the serious accident he had had with his truck, even though he had gotten a severe cut on his leg. After he lost his trucking job and was penniless, he had ended up at the Salvation Army in Chicago, but they had realized immediately that he was different. They knew he was not the average "slum-bum" that they were used to. I will always be grateful that they were kind and considerate. They counseled him to go back to his family, and that is what he finally did.

We felt that the Lord had been watching over him and now he was where we could watch over him. He had made it back for my graduation from nursing.

After I graduated I worked at Loma Linda for a couple of years. As I think it over, it seems to me that Daddy started getting sick just when Jacquee and I most needed his help and guidance in our life decisions. When I had dates, often they would inquire, "What really is the problem with your father?"

The doctors were still giving us vague answers.

I sometimes sit and think about Daddy—how strong he was when I was a little girl. I can hear him preaching. I can hear him laughing. His personality was so vivacious. He was such a beautiful person in every way.

When he began to get sick, and his face and mouth began twitching and moving all the time, I know now that he was embarrassed and knew that something was wrong with him, but there seemed no way to find out what it was.

I met my husband while I was working and teaching at Loma Linda. Since Jacquee had decided to remarry, we hit upon the idea of a double wedding. It was really very special to both of us. Daddy was well enough to walk down the aisle with one of us on each arm. Most of our family was there.

My own husband has been the most helpful, kindest, and loving of Christian companions to me and has understood my grief over my father.

Our first child, Becky, was born while we still lived in

Loma Linda. Daddy was thrilled with her. He called her his "Easter bunny" because she was born on Easter Sunday morning. I think he missed her terribly when we moved to the Midwest, but this was a good opportunity for my husband. I, though, was very lonely for Daddy and Mother and was so happy to see them when she brought him on a trip when our little boy was born.

How I wished that I had lived near enough so that they could have dropped in at any time. It would have been so much better for Mother. How I wish also that I could have helped Mother with Daddy's care, for it was so strenuous.

The last time Mother brought Daddy to see us, after we had moved to Denver, they put him on the airplane before anyone else and then kept him and Mother until everyone else had gotten off and put him in a motorized cart to bring him to where we were waiting for him. The problem was that as his disease progressed, he could not control his muscles, and so his legs would spasm. To make any progress he would have to sort of shuffle along, and rock from side to side.

Also the muscles in his throat would twitch and spasm. His speech was terribly affected. He almost blurted out his words explosively, or he could not talk at all. He had always enjoyed eating when he was well, but as his sickness got worse, he became terribly thin, which is characteristic of H.D. It took a very long time for him to eat a meal, for he had more and more problems with swallowing. He could not control the muscles in his throat. Often he would cough and choke, and in the final stages of his illness this terrified him, for he had the sensation of choking to death and suffocating, over and over.

Mother would make milkshakes for him, putting in all the nutritious elements she could think of. He would drink these with a straw, and that worked better.

When my sister and I were growing up, I remember that Daddy always thanked Mother for the meals she prepared. He always said, "Thank you, Snooksie (or "Precious Little

Mommy"), for the wonderful meal"—even when Mother didn't think she'd fixed anything very great and I guess sometimes we girls didn't either! And when Daddy got so he couldn't swallow very well and Mother would fix him the milkshakes, he would try to say "Thank you" as he had always done. It was so sad.

The year before he died was so hard, so hard. He had to have constant, twenty-four-hour-a-day care. When my sister and I realized that the end was near, we began to worry about Mother. Her whole life had been built around him for so long. She had literally thought of nothing else. She had been under such a constant strain for so many years. She had had to make all the decisions for him, for his welfare, for herself; financial decisions, career decisions—it was all up to her.

The hardest thing for all of us was to watch him getting thinner every day, his muscles in constant spasm, his whole body in agony, and to know that there was absolutely nothing that could be done to reverse the progress of the disease. We had not had any close family member die before, and I wondered whether we would be brave enough to face it all. My husband and I saved money all that last year for the trip we knew we would have to take to California. I didn't feel that I could talk to anyone in Denver about it, for I didn't want to try to explain all the aspects and tragedies of his disease. So I more or less stayed to myself, wondering what day I would get the phone call that he was gone, that my Daddy was dead. For that entire last year it seemed to me that I had a lump in my throat.

When finally the call came from Mother, in the early hours of the morning, it was really a relief to be able to fly to her and know that Daddy's long sufferings were over. Mother held herself together amazingly well. She had grown very close to God, becoming totally dependent on Him.

I have never felt closer to Christ than at the funeral. Daddy looked better in his casket than he had for so many, many years. Jacquee put a small Bible and Mother a tiny

United States flag in his hands, since he had enjoyed working in the religious liberty department so much. She also placed one red rose on the Bible, symbolizing the many beautiful roses he had given her during their happy years.

I can hardly wait until Jesus comes and puts an end to all the sorrow and sickness and suffering in the world. My children will have a chance to know the grandfather that they have been deprived of, one who will run and play with them and teach them about the animals and stars that he loved.

The theme of Daddy's life, I believe, was the love of Jesus, the love that He has for each one of us, how much He cares for us. That was what he liked most to preach about as I was growing up. I have seen this love manifested in my mother's behalf. In spite of all that she has gone through, in spite of all the tears and anguish, she is her old self again, vivacious and full of plans for the future.

APPENDIX C
Stanley

STANLEY MARSHALL BUCK was born on October 19, 1916, the third son of Claude and Margaret Buck. While his mother carried him she contracted tuberculosis. As a result, she wondered whether she would survive, and whether the new baby would survive. When it was time for her delivery, a friend drove her to the hospital.

"If I don't live, will you take the baby?" she begged her friend. "I don't think Claude could manage any other way. After all, the other boys are only 4 and 2," she continued.

But Margaret Buck lived to leave the hospital in Sacramento and to take home small Stanley. However, she was so weak, so unable to do the heavy work of the household, that Claude's sister, Ruth, made her home with them. From the first days of his life, Stanley regarded Ruth as his mother; she was the person who cared for him, bathed him, fed him, and watched over him.

As Stanley's mother became conscious that the end for her was very near, again she tried to make provisions for the small child. "Ruth, Stanley is just like your own baby. You have cared for him since his birth. When I am gone, please take him as your own."

By this time Ruth loved him as a mother would, though she was not married and did not have her own home. But she could not give him up. She returned to her parents' home in Rio Linda, a small town north of Sacramento. Little Stanley was the center of her existence. Later, when a neighboring rancher, Wilton Jefferson, asked her to be his wife, it was understood that Stanley would be part of the new home.

The ranch life provided a wonderful home for the tiny boy right from the beginning, marred only by a bout with pneumonia that almost cost him his life. Ruth ("Mother" to him) worked ceaselessly night and day with fomentations and other treatments. Finally the crisis passed.

As the years passed no attempt was ever made to keep the knowledge of his natural father and brothers from Stanley. He learned that his father had never been physically strong and that he had no interest in Adventism. His mother, an Adventist, had longed for at least one of her sons to be brought up in this faith, though her own background was Christian Science.

Probably because of the novelty of knowing he had "another father" and two older brothers, Stanley as a child cherished the few contacts that developed. On the rare occasions when he was with them, he seemed to feel that he "belonged," and suffered small feelings of bereavement when they separated. Stan's "real" father drifted from religion to religion, and eventually died when Stan was already a young minister. The first time, however, that Stan spoke in the Modesto, California, church after he had been elected to the religious liberty department of the Pacific Union, his real father came to hear him and sat on the front row, tears streaming down his proud face. Stan's older brother was killed in Oregon when only about 16, but Stan kept in contact with Robert, his other brother, and during Stan's illness Robert was a strength and comfort to him.

Ruth and Wilton Jefferson were, to all intents and purposes, his parents, and certainly they were the strongest influence in his developmental years. They loved him devotedly, along with a daughter later born to them. When Stanley was about 9 years old, Mr. Jefferson felt a strong call from the Lord to become a singing evangelist. At that time it was not unusual for men to enter the ministry via routes other than college training; it was thought by some that these men might indeed have stronger convictions and do a greater work for God than others.

After the ranch had been sold and Wilton Jefferson had entered the work, he took his family to Pacific Union College while he took a short course of study. Then the family traveled from tent effort to tent effort in northern California. Stan attended a number of church schools, graduating from the eighth grade at Roseville and from Golden Gate Academy in Oakland.

When Stan entered Pacific Union College in 1935, Father Jefferson was in pastoral work in southern California, having been successful in this phase of the ministry for some time. Prior to this, Stanley had grown into a very enterprising teen-ager, running a small "bread route" for a woman who launched into a homemade bread project and doing other kinds of selling. He had been able in his late teens actually to buy a little dilapidated car that he kept running. Few teen-agers in that time period owned cars.

During those days of the great depression and its aftermath, Stanley was considered by his peers to be somewhat better off than the average young college student.

Because he never knew his natural mother, and did not learn anything about her family until he was an adult, he never ascertained the source of the fatal gene that carried the dread disease of Huntington's chorea.